Advance Praise for *Sumo for Mixed Martial Arts*

"I recommend this *Sumo for Mixed Martial Arts* book to those who want to improve their grappling."

—Lyoto "The Dragon" Machida, Former UFC light heavyweight champion

"Andrew Zerling is clearly a man with an unmistakable passion for both sumo and MMA, armed with an acute awareness of how to best incorporate the culture and techniques of the ancient Japanese sport into the world of modern day MMA. A valuable addition to the library of anyone with an interest in either sumo or MMA—or both."

—Mark A. Buckton, Sumo writer, *Japan Times,*
Editor-in-chief, *Hello Japan, Tokyo & Capital Getaways*

"Andrew Zerling has done us all a service by taking what has been commonly regarded as a compartmentalized martial sport, sumo, and allowing us a peek inside its history and principles and giving us the opportunity to see how rich this vein of information can be to inform the modern incarnation of MMA."

—Mark Hatmaker, Best-selling author of thirteen titles including
the *No Holds Barred Fighting* series

"To me, sumo is the earliest codified form of jujitsu. It's the original art of distraction, angles, and leverage, seeking victory through the initial off balancing of an opponent. It's not necessary to throw your opponent cleanly on his back, as they do in judo, or force him to quit with a submission hold, as they do in Brazilian jiu-jitsu. These are the modern branches of jujitsu, while sumo is the root. The techniques of sumo are of benefit to all martial artists, particularly in the clinch and takedown phases, and are even easier to utilize against opponents in your own weight class in competition. *Sumo for Mixed Martial Arts: Winning Clinches, Takedowns, and Tactics* by Andrew Zerling is for serious students who want to evolve their grappling skills in mixed martial arts through a mindful look at the past. Taking the best of what has gone before allows us to create a vibrant, adaptive future and is always worthy of exploration."

—Roy Dean, Aikikai aikido black belt, Kodokan judo black belt, Brazilian
jiu-jitsu second-degree black belt, Seibukan jujitsu third-degree black belt

"During the time I was publishing the *Journal of Asian Martial Arts* (1992–2012), Andrew Zerling had submitted a number of articles for possible publication in our quarterly. Three were dealing with formidable submission techniques, which were analyzed, discussed, and demonstrated by Renzo Gracie and himself. All three articles were soon published, as each represented no-nonsense grappling and was presented with an authority derived from realistic hands-on experience.

"From his articles, e-mails, and phone conversations, it was apparent that Zerling was a stickler for details. Perhaps his bachelor of science degree in biology from Temple University and experience working as a technical writer for the food and drug industry equipped him with a keen eye and the drive to pursue logical conclusions. Such research skills coupled with an inquiring mind led him to make novel connections for the place sumo has in the wider range of combative techniques, particularly applicable in today's mixed martial arts (MMA).

"The last journal we published in 2012 included Zerling's article titled 'Sumo Wrestling: Practical Techniques for the Martial Artist' (*Journal of Asian Martial Arts, 21*[1]: 102–119). His thought process is outside the normal box of combative research! The article was well received, and Zerling was inspired to dive further into research to see what gems existed in traditional sumo techniques that could be applied in MMA. Because of his dedication fueled by scientific inquiry, he produced this book, from which all martial art practitioners can now benefit.

"The techniques and tactics presented are derived from a fine selection of case studies made by Zerling, supported by his viewing of sumo competitions, including the live tournament in Osaka, Japan. Zerling has wrenched information from his years of combative studies to benefit your own perception and practice—something you'll have fun incorporating."

   —**Michael DeMarco**, Publisher, Via Media Publishing Company

"I am so pleased that Andrew Zerling has written his outstanding book, *Sumo for Mixed Martial Arts*. I have been a fan of sumo technique since my first exposure to top sumotori in Japan in the mid-nineties. It takes extremely precise technique and effective tactics for one huge athlete to throw another gigantic, highly trained competitor. Anyone interested in combative sports or self-defense would be wise to explore the methods of sumo, and Mr. Zerling's book is the perfect entrée."

   —**Burton Richardson**, Author, *Silat for the Street, Choke 'Em Out, JKD Unlimited, In the Footsteps of Bruce Lee, Black Belt Magazine* Self-Defense Instructor of the Year, 2015, Black Belt Hall of Fame

"I find the correlation, comparisons, and similarities between grappling styles and cultural origins fascinating. This is a captivating book, well researched and thought out, truly enlightening for all who love the grappling arts."

   —**Chris Haueter**, Brazilian jiu-jitsu fifth-degree black belt

"The ancient art of sumo isn't about four-hundred-pound mountains of flesh smashing into one another but rather a sophisticated fighting art based on precise timing and well-honed techniques. Andrew Zerling's unique and information-crammed *Sumo for Mixed Martial Arts* uses high-quality pics and easy-to-follow instruction, guaranteed to take your up-close-and-personal fighting skill to the next level."

   —**Loren W. Christensen**, Author and veteran martial artist

"*Sumo for Mixed Martial Arts: Winning Clinches, Takedowns, and Tactics* offers another tool to protect oneself or survive if engaged in hand-to-hand combat. The book rightly deserves a place on the bookshelf of martial arts enthusiasts."

—**Robert S. Fiero, Col. USA (Ret.)**, Coauthor, *Conquering Fear* and *Power of Courage in Combat and Danger*

"As a coach, practitioner, and fan of another esoteric grappling art (catch-as-catch-can), I was thrilled to read Andrew Zerling's *Sumo for Mixed Martial Arts*. Zerling's historical and technical exposition shows sumo to be both palpable and relevant for today's athletes engaged in the sport of mixed martial arts. What a fascinating read!"

—**Jake Shannon**, Author, *Say Uncle!: Catch-As-Catch-Can Wrestling and the Roots of Ultimate Fighting, Pro Wrestling, & Modern Grappling,* Coauthor, *Physical Chess: My Life in Catch-As-Catch-Can Wrestling*

"Andrew Zerling's *Sumo For Mixed Martial Arts* is a well-written and thoroughly researched book that draws attention to a martial art that is seldom taken seriously outside of Japan—and one that is certainly not part of most fighters' training repertoire. Hopefully, this book will go some way towards seeing the adoption of sumo as a practical grappling art within the cage and help it to gain the recognition it deserves."

—**Neal Molyneaux**, Managing editor, *MMA Uncaged Magazine*

"Andrew Zerling is not only a very methodical researcher and writer, but a man who actually gets in the ring and puts his words into practice. The collection of photographs which sequentially show how to adapt the techniques to an MMA situation is worth its weight in gold. I like the way he has focused on distinctive wrestlers who clearly embody their respective sumo fighting styles. An accessible read which should prove of real practical value to anyone seeking to broaden their knowledge of possible MMA techniques."

—**Chris Gould**, Author, *Sumo through the Wrestlers' Eyes*, *Sumo's Strongest Men*, and *Sumo: Amateur versus Professional*

"*Sumo for Mixed Martial Arts: Winning Clinches, Takedowns, and Tactics* is a great read. This well-researched book presented by Andrew Zerling delves into the roots of jujitsu, focusing on the discipline's original self-defense emphasis and its subsequent adaptation for sport fighting as applicable to sumo. I appreciated many of Andrew's sport-fighting insights, particularly those involving the practical importance of sumo open-handed strikes, the importance of always moving and remaining on the balls of one's feet, and, of course, that the best defense is a good offense. One quote also had particular resonance for both sport and street fighting: 'To do something illegal in a fighter's game, something he doesn't know, is the best way to beat any fighter.' This superb commentary obviously has street-defense applications as well. I encourage any mixed martial artist or fighting sports enthusiast to read this rewarding book."

—**David Kahn**, Author, *Krav Maga, Advanced Krav Maga, Krav Maga Weapon Defenses, Krav Maga Professional Tactics*, and *Krav Maga Defense*

"*Sumo for Mixed Martial Arts* is part history, part case study, and part technical instruction. It introduces the reader to the application of ancient sumo techniques and strategies, and applies them to modern mixed martial arts. Careful study of favorite techniques of both previous sumo masters and modern MMA fighters offers a fascinating insight into their styles. The manual finishes with detailed explanations and photographs of more than forty techniques, including throws, locks, trips, sweeps, pushes, and strikes. Taken together, the book delivers a unique blend of historical study and practical application that simply cannot be found elsewhere."

—**Dr. Arthur T. Bradley**, Kenpo karate second-degree black belt, Author, *The Survivalist* series, *Handbook to Practical Disaster: Preparedness for the Family, The Prepper's Instruction Manual, Disaster Preparedness for EMP Attacks and Solar Storms*, and *Process of Elimination*

"*Sumo for Mixed Martial Arts* is a fascinating insight into an often misunderstood area of martial arts. Most people are aware of the sumo style, but few have examined its techniques and strategies in detail, especially in regard to modern mixed martial arts combat.

"Zerling has explored the colorful, surprising history of sumo and extracted an engaging, practical set of theories on the application of grappling, clinching, and more for the modern combatant.

"In an age when Brazilian jiu-jitsu and muay Thai seem to be de rigueur within MMA, this book takes a fresh look at training and asks *what if there is another way?* Fascinating reading for any martial arts fan."

—**Phil Pierce**, Bestselling author, *Martial Arts: Behind the Myths* and *Self Defense Made Simple,* Creator of BlackBeltFit.com

"I have been studying martial arts for over thirty-five years and have been introduced to many styles from all over the world. I have a huge passion for Japanese martial arts, which brought me to study judo, karate, kendo, and iaido for many years. Being involved in these arts exposed me to the art of sumo. It has always been fascinating to me to watch such large athletes move so quickly, with such agility and surprising flexibility.

"Many people look at sumo as a clash of giants, which at a quick glance, it is. But what most don't realize is that it is actually a sport of speed, timing, leverage, and strategy.

"Being able to use an opponent's size and strength against them takes a great understanding of body mechanics, leverage, and a chess-like mind-set, where you have to think a few steps ahead to get your opponent to move the way you want in order to take them down.

"This is very similar to many grappling arts where skill beats strength. In catch wrestling and MMA, being able to use the clinch effectively can easily change the outcome of a fight. If things aren't going your way at long range, you need to be able to close the distance and engage in a tie-up and eventually set up a takedown. Andrew does an excellent job of illustrating this in *Sumo for MMA*. As a catch wrestler and coach to high-level MMA fighters, I can appreciate the strategy and clinch work of sumo. It can easily be applied to the ring or cage, as you will see in the many techniques found in this book."

> —**John Potenza**, Cofounder, Snake Pit U.S.A. Catch Wrestling Association, Combat Submission Wrestling representative instructor, MMA and muay Thai coach, Martial artist since 1981

"This text balances instruction with deep insights, giving mixed martial artists the understanding and skills they need to excel.

"*Sumo for Mixed Martial Arts: Winning Clinches, Takedowns, and Tactics* by Andrew Zerling equips practitioners of other martial arts to add sumo to their skill set.

"Early portions of the book focus on the history, culture, and significance of sumo wrestling. Zerling immediately goes far beyond the simple stereotypes and cartoonish notions that most people—even many martial artists—may hold related to this less-practiced craft. This depth and background is shown to be necessary for understanding any martial art, and helps the text balance attention on the importance of thinking as well as of doing.

"It may be tempting to jump to the technical photos later in the book, but Zerling reveals that every fighter needs to fully understand their martial art in order to do it well. He paces the introduction nicely, keeping martial artists engaged and ensuring that they will have room to grasp key concepts before proceeding. The third chapter, which links sumo and mixed martial arts, ties together the background, what mixed martial artists already know, and the practical skills that come later in the book. Once the book gets to the instructional section, which fills the bulk of the pages, Zerling's approach turns to no-nonsense action and instruction, showcasing skills that fighters can apply on the mat right away.

"Zerling is a black belt with several decades of experience in a number of martial arts. His expertise and interdisciplinary approach shine through in the book's balance of instruction and depth of insight. His background as a technical writer is also apparent in the book's straightforward, thorough, and no-frills prose.

"Zerling's key audience is experienced mixed martial artists who want to add depth and complexity to their fighting repertoire through sumo. The book is best suited for those who take their craft seriously and who want to grow in skill as well as in understanding, but who have little or no experience with sumo. Those new to mixed martial arts will find this book inspiring, but not as practically useful as it is for those with more skills or experience.

"The numerous step-by-step photos are a key feature of the book. These serve as a guide through the sport's complex actions, helping to show how motions operate, even when single photos can't fully encapsulate motion and direction. Occasionally the images run small, but experienced fighters will have the confidence and know-how to understand and apply what they see.

"*Sumo for Mixed Martial Arts* is a thoughtful work that will help to make mixed martial artists more centered and formidable in their craft."

—**Melissa Wuske**, *Foreword Reviews*

SUMO

FOR Mixed Martial Arts

Winning Clinches, Takedowns, and Tactics

ANDREW ZERLING

YMAA Publication Center, Inc.
Wolfeboro, NH USA

YMAA Publication Center, Inc.
PO Box 480
Wolfeboro, New Hampshire, 03894
1-800-669-8892 • info@ymaa.com • www.ymaa.com

ISBN: 9781594394096 (print) • ISBN: 9781594394102 (ebook)

Edited by Doran Hunter
Cover design by Axie Breen
Photos by Kristopher Schoenleber unless noted otherwise
This book typeset in 12 pt. Adobe Garamond.

10   9   8   7   6   5   4   3   2   1

Publisher's Cataloging in Publication

Names: Zerling, Andrew,
Title: Sumo for mixed martial arts : winning clinches, takedowns, and tactics / Andrew Zerling.
Description: Wolfeboro, New Hampshire : YMAA Publication Center, Inc., [2016] | Includes bibliographical
    references.
Identifiers: ISBN: 978-1-59439-355-6 (print) | 978-1-59439-356-3 (ebook) | LCCN: 2016952681
Subjects: LCSH: Mixed martial arts—Handbooks, manuals, etc. | Mixed martial arts—Technique. | Sumo—
    Technique. | Wrestling—Technique. | Wrestling--Takedown. | Hand-to-hand fighting, Oriental—Throws. |
    Judo—Throws. | Martial arts—Technique. | BISAC: SPORTS & RECREATION / Martial Arts & Self-
    Defense. | HEALTH & FITNESS / Exercise.
Classification: LCC: GV1102.7.M59 Z47 2016 | DDC: 796.815—dc23

Editorial note: In Japanese tradition, the family name precedes a person's given name—that is, the "last name" comes first. English-language publishers often reverse these names for the benefit of their readers. For example, while the Japanese may speak of Funakoshi Gichin, many Western readers know him as Gichin Funakoshi. We have observed the Western style in this book.

The authors and publisher of the material are NOT RESPONSIBLE in any manner whatsoever for any injury that may occur through reading or following the instructions in this manual.

The activities, physical or otherwise, described in this manual may be too strenuous or dangerous for some people, and the reader(s) should consult a physician before engaging in them.

Warning: While self-defense is legal, fighting is illegal. If you don't know the difference, you'll go to jail because you aren't defending yourself. You are fighting—or worse. Readers are encouraged to be aware of all appropriate local and national laws relating to self-defense, reasonable force, and the use of weaponry, and to act in accordance with all applicable laws at all times. Understand that while legal definitions and interpretations are generally uniform, there are small—but very important—differences from state to state and even city to city. To stay out of jail, you need to know these differences. Neither the author nor the publisher assumes any responsibility for the use or misuse of information contained in this book.

Nothing in this document constitutes a legal opinion, nor should any of its contents be treated as such. While the author believes everything herein is accurate, any questions regarding specific self-defense situations, legal liability, and/or interpretation of federal, state, or local laws should always be addressed by an attorney at law.

When it comes to martial arts, self-defense, and related topics, no text, no matter how well written, can substitute for professional hands-on instruction. These materials should be used for academic study only.

Printed in Canada.

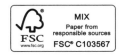

Contents

Foreword by Steve Scott   xiii

Foreword by Stephan Kesting   xv

Preface   xvii

Acknowledgments   xix

CHAPTER 1—Sumo Wrestling Overview   1
    Introduction   1
    Sumo History and Practice   4
    Sumo vs. Other Japanese Martial Arts   8
    Professional vs. Amateur Sumo   9
    Sumo's Winning Moves   10
    Overview Conclusion   12

CHAPTER 2—Sumo Wrestling Case Studies   13
    Introduction   13
    Case Study 1: Mainoumi—"Department Store of Techniques"   13
    Case Study 2: Akebono—Grand Champion, Yokozuna   16
    Case Study 3: Konishiki—Ozeki "Meat Bomb"   17
    Case Study 4: Terao—"Iron Man" of Sumo   18
    Case Study 5: Open-Hand Attacks   19
    Case Study 6: Dominating Techniques   21
    Case Studies Conclusion   23

CHAPTER 3—Sumo and MMA   25
    Introduction   25
    The Clinch Phase   26
    The Over-Under Clinch   27
    Why the Takedown?   29
    The Complete MMA Fighter   31
    Mitsuyo "Count Trouble" Maeda: Father of Brazilian Jiu-Jitsu   33
    Lyoto "The Dragon" Machida: Former UFC LHW Champion   35
    David vs. Goliath   37
    Physical Conditioning   40
    Sumo and MMA Conclusion   41

CHAPTER 4—Technical Photos 43

Introduction 43

Breakfalls (Ukemi) 43

Forward Breakfall (Mae Ukemi) 44

Rear Breakfall (Ushiro Ukemi) 46

Side Breakfall (Yoko Ukemi) 48

Forward-Rolling Breakfall (Mae Mawari Ukemi) 50

Sumo and MMA Fighting Stances 51

Sumo Fighting Stance 52

MMA Fighting Stance 52

Supplementary Techniques 53

Grips 53

Over-Under Clinch 54

Underhook Technique 55

Over-Under Clinch Exercise 56

Push Escape from the Over-Under Clinch 57

Push Escape from the Double-Underhooks Clinch, Two Ways 58

Kimarite: Sumo's Winning Moves 60

Basic Techniques (Kihonwaza) 60

Front Push Out (Oshidashi) 61

Front Push Down (Oshitaoshi) 62

Front Thrust Out (Tsukidashi) 64

Front Thrust Down (Tsukitaoshi) 66

Throwing Techniques (Nagete) 68

One-Arm Shoulder Throw (Ipponzeoi) 68

Hooking Inner-Thigh Throw (Kakenage) 70

Hip Throw (Koshinage) 71

Armlock Throw (Kotenage) 72

Headlock Throw (Kubinage) 74

Body-Drop Throw (Nichonage) 76

Beltless Arm Throw (Sukuinage) 78

Inner-Thigh-Lift Throw (Yaguranage) 80

Leg-Tripping Techniques (Kakete) 82

Leg Pick (Ashitori) 82

Pulling Heel Hook (Chongake) 84

Inside Foot Sweep (Kekaeshi) 85

Twisting Backward Knee Trip (Kirikaeshi) 86

Inside Thigh Scoop (Komatasukui) 88

Triple-Attack Force Out (Mitokorozeme) 90

Ankle-Sweep Twist Down (Nimaigeri) 92

Outside Leg Trip (Sotogake) 94

Outside Thigh Scoop (Sotokomata) 96

Rear Foot Sweep (Susoharai) 98

Ankle Pick (Susotori) 100

Inside Leg Trip (Uchigake)   102
Thigh-Grabbing Push Down (Watashikomi)   104
Twist-Down Techniques (Hinerite)   106
Fisherman's Throw (Amiuchi)   106
Clasped-Hand Twist Down (Gasshohineri)   108
Two-Handed Arm Twist Down (Kainahineri)   110
Under-Shoulder Swing Down (Katasukashi)   112
Armlock Twist Down (Kotehineri)   114
Head-Twisting Throw (Kubihineri)   116
Twist Down (Makiotoshi)   118
Outer-Thigh-Sweep Twist Down (Sotomuso)   120
Two-Handed Head Twist Down (Tokkurinage)   122
Armbar Throw (Tottari)   124
Armbar-Throw Counter (Sakatottari)   126
Thrust Down Forward (Tsukiotoshi)   128
Inner-Thigh-Sweep Twist Down (Uchimuso)   130
Head-Pivot Throw (Zubuneri)   132
Special Techniques (Tokushuwaza)   134
Slap Down (Hatakikomi)   134
Hand Pull Down (Hikiotoshi)   136
Arm-Pull Force Out (Hikkake)   138
Armbar Force Down (Kimetaoshi)   140
Rear Leg Trip (Okurigake)   142
Rear Pull Down (Okurihikiotoshi)   144
Rear Throw Down (Okurinage)   146
Rear-Lift Body Slam (Okuritsuriotoshi)   148
Head Slap Down (Sokubiotoshi)   150
Conclusion   151

Bibliography   153

Notes   155

Index   157

About the Author   163

Preface

After witnessing a live professional grand sumo tournament in Japan, I became even more enthralled by this well-known but misunderstood martial art. The barrel-like physique of the sumo wrestler contrasts strikingly with the lean, muscular physique of the average combat sports athlete. Because of this, many see sumo as spectacle devoid of real athleticism. But make no mistake: professional sumo wrestlers are easily on par with Olympic-level athletes.

When I explored sumo more carefully, I found that it is just as deeply technical a martial art as judo or Western wrestling. In applying its techniques to my own diverse grappling martial arts training, I have gained an even greater respect for this underestimated martial art. I wanted to share my insights with the martial arts community, so I wrote a seventeen-page academic article titled "Sumo Wrestling: Practical Techniques for the Martial Artist" that was published in the final issue of the *Journal of Asian Martial Arts*. The encouraging feedback spawned my idea of significantly expanding my sumo article and making it a book.

Clinches and takedowns are the most overlooked aspect of many martial artists' game. My book, *Sumo for Mixed Martial Arts: Winning Clinches, Takedowns, and Tactics*, solves this problem. Sumo wrestling's little-known but ancient proven clinches, takedowns, and tactics offer a fresh, new perspective. Martial artists who stand to benefit from this book include mixed martial arts (MMA) fighters, practitioners of all arts that involve grappling, self-defense practitioners, nongrappling martial artists, and serious sumo fans in general.

In this book, I first offer an overview of sumo wrestling. Second, we will examine sumo "case studies" to show in detail how a sumo wrestler can technically win a match. Third, we will take a close look at sumo from an MMA perspective. And finally, I will illustrate many sumo techniques relevant to MMA with photos—not line drawings—of actual martial artists performing them. This book is organized so the reader can progressively build on the information as it is presented in a logical order. To gain the most benefit, then, this book should be read from the beginning to the end.

The link between sumo and other martial arts has never before been deeply explored in a book. Brazilian jiu-jitsu and MMA are two of the fastest-growing sports in the world, and sumo has much to contribute to both. Many think they know what sumo is, but what they know is only the surface. This book goes far beyond the surface to uncover theory and techniques that can be of tremendous benefit to many martial artists. I sincerely hope this book brings sumo into the spotlight as a traditional and practical martial art to be studied by all types of martial artists.

—Andrew Zerling

Acknowledgments

To my family, friends, teachers, training partners, publishers, and proofreaders who assisted me in honing my martial arts skills, my writing skills, and most importantly, my life skills. For without your support, this book would not exist.

"If I have seen further it is by standing on the shoulders of giants."—Isaac Newton

I would like to thank my excellent training partners, Matthew Wavro and Davide Ballatori, for their invaluable assistance in demonstrating the techniques in this book. Special thanks to my professional photographer, Kristopher Schoenleber, for masterfully capturing these techniques with his dynamic photos.

CHAPTER 1

Sumo Wrestling Overview

Introduction

Suddenly after an intense staring contest, two huge men powerfully collide in an earthen ring. They are thickly muscled, flexible, highly trained martial artists; they are sumo wrestlers (*rikishi*). The initial collision of two rikishi can generate an incredible one ton of force or even more. All other things equal, the bigger rikishi usually wins. But rarely are all other things equal. Throughout sumo's history there have been smaller rikishi who, with the proper technique, have toppled mountain-like men. A sumo historian once said the earthen ring where sumo takes place (*dohyo*) is circular to help a smaller rikishi angle away from a larger rikishi. This allows for more interesting matches, and it also shows that in some ways, sumo roots for the underdog.

Japan's ancient and popular martial art is greatly overlooked in the West. This book focuses on sumo's winning moves, with special emphasis on how smaller players can win against larger players. Because sumo techniques allow a small rikishi to take down larger rikishi, there are clearly benefits in sumo for other martial arts, particularly in mixed martial arts (MMA) and other grappling arts. Modern MMA grew mostly out of jujitsu, and sumo can be seen as the root of jujitsu. Sumo, then, is ultimately one of the major roots of modern MMA. Sumo and modern MMA may look vastly different, but if it were not for the great technical fighting advancements of ancient sumo, there probably would be no MMA as we know it today.

Sumo wrestling predates jujitsu by many centuries.[1] Sumo goes back about fifteen hundred years, while the first recorded jujitsu school was not formed in Japan until about five hundred years ago. Considering that sumo was an integral part of the Japanese culture for many centuries before the numerous refined empty-hand techniques of jujitsu were introduced, it would be logical to think sumo had a strong influence in the development of jujitsu.

Sumo can been considered the earliest codified form of jujitsu. Many of the *kimarite*, sumo's winning moves, are similar to modern-day jujitsu and judo techniques. They also have similar names. Sumo's one-arm shoulder throw, *ipponzeoi,* has a counterpart in jujitsu's full shoulder throw called *ippon seoi nage.* Sumo's *koshinage,* a hip throw, is similar to jujitsu's *o-goshi* or full hip throw, and the same goes for *sotogake,* sumo's outside leg trip, and jujitsu's *kosoto-gake,* or small outer hook.

Sumo can be seen as one of the oldest and most primal and powerful of the Japanese martial arts. So it is not hard to understand why we may view sumo as the root of jujitsu. Some other martial arts, such as judo, aikido, and Brazilian jiu-jitsu (BJJ), are all modern-day forms of jujitsu,[2] each having different objectives and associated techniques that have changed over time to coincide with those objectives.

Some well-known martial artists have studied sumo. The founder of judo, Jigoro Kano, studied not only jujitsu but also a great variety of martial arts, including sumo, to help formulate his modern-day judo.[3] When Kano wanted to beat a competitor, he would study everything available, along with sumo techniques and even training books from abroad. Early on, Kano used his knowledge of a sumo shoulder-throw technique to help him create the shoulder-wheel throw (*kata-guruma*), which is similar to Western wrestling's fireman's carry. He used this new throw to defeat a tough opponent. Kano collected nearly one hundred transmission scrolls (texts containing the secrets of the system) from many different schools of martial arts, including sumo.[4]

In Okinawa, karate master and pioneer Gichin Funakoshi in his youth engaged in sumo-like wrestling called *tegumi,* which he recounts in his book *Karate-Do, My Way of Life.* Funakoshi mentioned in his book that he cannot be sure how much tegumi helped his karate mastery, but it definitely had a positive impact. His tegumi training helped him gain muscular strength, which is very beneficial in karate. Also, Funakoshi is certain that tegumi assisted in fortifying his will, an attribute every martial artist needs.[5] Tegumi branched off in two directions: the self-defense version, karate, and the sport version, Okinawan sumo. Hence, many Okinawan karate masters also practiced tegumi.

The founder of aikido, Morihei Ueshiba, started his first real training in the martial arts with sumo. In *Abundant Peace*, Stevens describes the grueling conditioning Ueshiba endured during his sumo training. Even while in the Imperial Army as a young man, Ueshiba was still remarkable at sumo. Ueshiba's early training in sumo, which focused "on keeping one's center of gravity low," probably had an influence on the development of aikido in his later years.[6] All three profoundly influential martial arts masters, Kano (1860–1938), Funakoshi (1868–1957), and Ueshiba (1883–1969) saw the great importance of adding sumo to their martial arts training routine.[7]

More recently, former UFC Light Heavyweight Champion Lyoto Machida, besides being an expert in Shotokan karate and BJJ, has a strong background in sumo. Machida describes in his book *Machida Karate-Do Mixed Martial Arts Techniques* that his sumo training strengthened his fighting stance and base, as well as his mind.[8] With his open-minded approach to martial arts training, Machida has become one of the most formidable MMA fighters of his time. Later in this book we will examine his fighting style in depth, especially his outstanding use of sumo techniques and tactics in MMA competition. Even in the modern arena of MMA, Machida saw the value of integrating some sumo into his MMA fighting game.

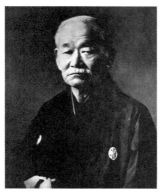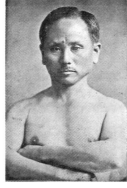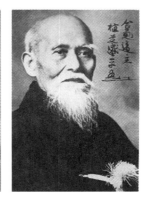

All three profoundly influential martial arts masters, Kano (1860–1938), Funakoshi (1868–1957), and Ueshiba (1883–1969), saw the great importance of adding sumo to their martial arts training routine.

(Left: Kano, courtesy of Uchina, Wikimedia Commons. Middle: Funakoshi, courtesy of Gichin Funakoshi, Wikimedia Commons. Right: Ueshiba, courtesy of Sakurambo, Wikimedia Commons.)

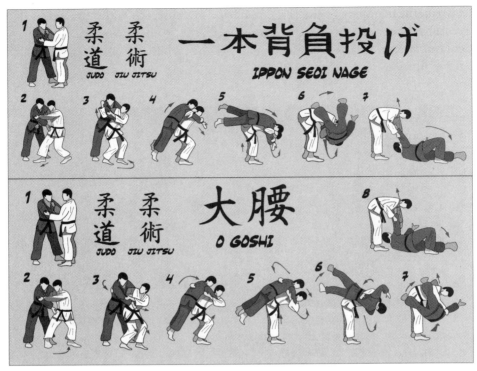

The judo/jujitsu throws full shoulder throw (ippon seoi nage) and full hip throw (o-goshi) have practically the same technique and name as its sumo kimarite counterparts one-arm shoulder throw (ipponzeoi) and hip throw (koshinage). This shows that there is a very close historical link between sumo and judo/jujitsu. There are numerous other instances of this connection—so much so that sumo could be considered the earliest codified form of judo/jujitsu.

(Upper: Ippon Seoi Nage, courtesy of bimserd, Can Stock Photo. Lower: O-Goshi, courtesy of bimserd, Can Stock Photo.)

Sumo History and Practice

Myth surrounds much of sumo's early history. It was a violent sumo match between the gods, it is said, that created the Japanese islands themselves. Sumo's Japanese beginnings go back about one thousand five hundred years, making sumo one of the oldest organized sports on earth. There is evidence that the precursors of the combat sport probably came from China or Korea. The earliest known record of sumo in Japan is its ancient predecessor known as *sumai*, which was practiced in a no-holds-barred wrestling style. Warlike sumai evolved to a more sportive sumo style of wrestling. Sumo essentially took its present style in the Edo period (AD 1603–1867).

In Japan, the first sumo matches were in religious ceremonies to pray for a good harvest, and eventually they were used as a training routine for samurai warriors. Masterless samurai warriors (*ronin*) even used their training in sumo matches as a way to earn extra money. Sumo had an influence in the development of many modern Japanese martial arts, and today it is the unofficial national sport of Japan. The complex system of rituals and etiquette of sumo are uniquely Japanese. It is significantly more than just two huge men wrestling. Even in modern Japanese society, rikishi are thought of as godlike heroes. Rikishi literally means "powerful man."

The rules of Japan's ancient martial art are not complex: the wrestler loses when he touches anything outside the ring before his opponent or when he first touches the surface inside the ring with something other than the soles of his feet. The outcome is decided in a short time (in seconds, rarely in minutes). In a small ring, in those seconds, the rikishi push themselves to the maximum, both mentally and physically.

The following are prohibited techniques in today's sumo matches and result in loss of a match due to disqualification:

- striking the opponent with a closed fist
- bending back one or more of the opponent's fingers
- grabbing the opponent's hair
- grabbing the opponent's throat
- jabbing at the opponent's eyes or solar plexus
- palm striking both of the opponent's ears at the same time
- grabbing or pulling at the opponent's groin area
- kicking at the opponent's chest or waist

Besides the disqualifying moves listed above, almost anything else is permitted to win a match.

Before a rikishi steps onto the dohyo for a major match, he must endure much rigorous and grueling training. The young rikishi train in a sumostable under the guidance of the stablemaster and his seniors. Young rikishi live in the stable, and their training starts early in the morning with mostly basic movements. Strength, flexibility, and reflex exercises are performed countless times until they become second nature, as well as breakfalls (*ukemi*), which protect them when they fall. Thigh splits (*matawari*) are an integral part of the daily training regimen to gain suppleness in the entire body. After going through the Japan Sumo Association training school, which lasts six months, a rikishi can sit down on the ground and perform a full split with his face and chest touching the ground. This is amazing conditioning, especially because the rikishi are well known for their monstrous power and explosiveness, not their flexibility.

Even the diet, a sort of sumo stew of fish, meat, and vegetables called *chanko-nabe*, is well calculated. This thick meal is rich in calories and protein when eaten with a lot of white rice so the rikishi can gain weight and keep it on. The schedule in which the rikishi train and eat is the key to how they put on weight. They train in the morning session on an empty stomach as the extreme workout requires, and at noon, famished, they eat as much chanko-nabe as they can. Then they take an afternoon nap to slow the food digestion so they can rapidly gain weight. The rikishi's physique is most efficient when it is bottom heavy, with a barrel stomach. This gives them a lower center of gravity, which makes it harder to be thrown or pushed out of the ring and also helps to keep opponents at a distance. The rikishi may appear fat, but because of their diet and intense exercise regimen they have a remarkable amount of muscle mass.

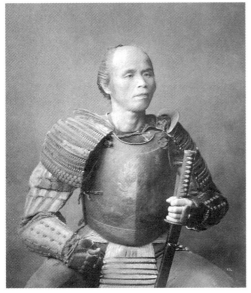

Samurai warrior, ca. 1877. In Japan, the first sumo matches were in religious ceremonies to pray for a good harvest, and eventually they were used as a training routine for samurai warriors.

(Library of Congress, LC-USZC4-14302.)

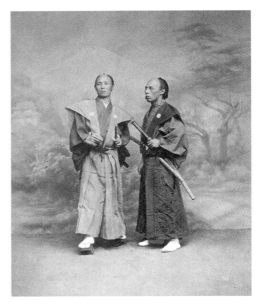

Two samurai warriors, ca. 1877. Masterless samurai warriors (ronin) even used their training in sumo matches as a way to earn extra money.

(Library of Congress, LC-USZC4-14305.)

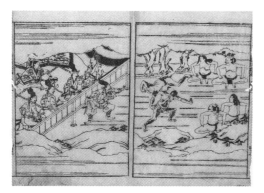

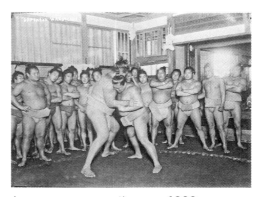

Japanese woodcut print of sumo wrestlers in action. Print created during the seventeenth century.
(Library of Congress, LC-DIG-jpd-02569.)

Japanese sumo wrestlers, ca. 1900.
(Library of Congress, LC-DIG-ggbain-26753.)

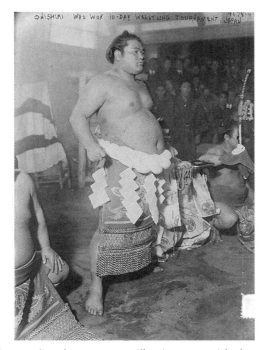

Onishiki (1891–1941) won a ten-day sumo wrestling tournament in Japan, ca. 1915. A bottom-heavy physique like Onishiki's makes it more difficult for the rikishi to be thrown or pushed out of the ring. Also, it helps keep the opponent at a distance.
(Library of Congress, LC-DIG-ggbain-24163.)

Sumo vs. Other Japanese Martial Arts

Professional sumo differs from other Japanese martial arts in the way that rank is awarded and maintained. In most other Japanese martial arts, rank is awarded by the successful completion of a ranking test. Rarely in the other Japanese martial arts is a practitioner demoted for continued bad competition results. Also, in other Japanese martial arts, promotion can be gained by other means of training, like forms (*kata*). With sumo, the rikishi is only promoted if he wins official tournament sumo matches and can easily be demoted if he loses them.

Rikishi who miss an official tournament through an injury will also be demoted badly. This forces some rikishi to wrestle with serious injuries. The rikishi's ability to win official tournament sumo matches, normally scheduled every two months, is the sole source of his livelihood and opportunity for promotion. The result is extremely stressful training and living conditions for the rikishi. This high-stress ranking structure could be seen as similar to the one in MMA competition. In MMA, if a fighter wins a championship belt, he will usually have to defend that belt or be demoted and therefore paid less, although MMA fighters tend to have fewer matches per year than a professional rikishi.

The strict hierarchy of sumo reflects traditional Japanese values. With higher rank come higher privileges. In sumo, it does not matter what your social status is; rank is achieved only through winning official tournament sumo matches. Grand Champion Akebono states, "If you want to understand sumo, you should watch the practice instead of the tournaments. In practice you can see what a difference ranking makes. It is what sumo life is based on."[9]

Also, most other martial arts competitions, especially the unarmed variety like karate, judo, and MMA, have weight divisions, unlike professional sumo. So it is not uncommon for a smaller rikishi to face a rikishi two times his size. This forces the smaller rikishi to be very technical in his fighting style to compensate. The soon-to-be-discussed rikishi Mainoumi is a prime example of this. Small but successful, he was well known for his very technical fighting style.

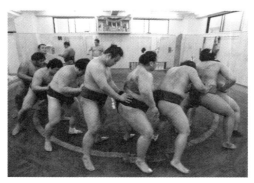

Unranked sumo wrestlers in training. On May 2, 1998, young unranked sumo wrestlers at the Tomozuma Stable in Tokyo end their daily workout routine with a ritualized dance that emphasizes teamwork.

(US Navy photo courtesy of M. Clayton Farrington, Wikimedia Commons.)

Professional vs. Amateur Sumo

There are many major distinctions between professional sumo and amateur sumo. Professional sumo is practiced only in Japan, while amateur sumo is mostly found in Japanese schools and to a lesser extent other parts of the world. Professional sumo has no weight divisions while amateur sumo does have weight divisions. Professional sumo is a way of life as compared to the part-time training in amateur sumo. The strength and skill in professional sumo is amazingly higher than in amateur sumo. Top amateurs would have trouble surviving against professional sumo's higher-division rikishi.

Professional sumo matches are always performed on a dohyo while amateur sumo matches many times take place on a simple matted surface. Also, females are allowed to compete in amateur sumo, but in professional sumo, not only are females not allowed to complete, but according to Japanese religious beliefs, females are also not even allowed to touch the dohyo as this will bring bad luck to the matches. And finally, much of the traditional sumo ceremony is gone from amateur sumo.

The dream of every young wrestler is to become yokozuna, *or grand champion. But most of those dreams will burst. . . . It's a very harsh world.*
—Wakamatsu Oyakata, sumo coach and elder[10]

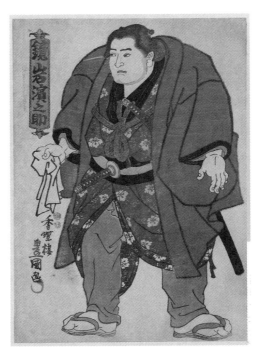

Print of sumo wrestler, ca. 1848. Notice that this rikishi carries two swords just as the samurai did. Sumo is closely linked to samurai tradition as can be seen with the use of the samurai topknot hairstyle in sumo tradition.

(Library of Congress, LC-DIG-jpd-00715.)

Sumo's Winning Moves

The winning moves in sumo are called kimarite. At this time, the Japan Sumo Association recognizes eighty-two types of kimarite, but only about a dozen are used regularly. In actuality more than half of sumo bouts end in victory after a push (*oshi*), grip (*yori*), or slap or thrust (*tsuki*). These eighty-two distinct winning moves include different combinations of gripping, pushing, thrusting, throwing, leg tripping, twist downs, backward body drops, and specialized moves. As stated earlier, kimarite are usually referred to as sumo's winning moves or finishing moves. In fact, at the end of a sumo match, an official will actually announce which kimarite was used to win the match.

Sumo's techniques were developed more than a thousand years ago. From the early Edo period (AD 1603–1867) there are lists that describe throws that still mirror many of the kimarite used today. The history of the kimarite goes back to the medieval Japanese era when there were the traditional forty-eight kimarite or *shijuuhatte* (forty-eight hands). However, in 1960 the Japan Sumo Association recognized a total of seventy kimarite. In the last three decades sumo has been internationalized in that a large percentage of rikishi in the top professional divisions are non-Japanese. The influx of foreign rikishi has influenced the techniques of sumo. Among the top influences are the following:

- The holds of folkstyle and Greco-Roman wrestling
- The charge of American football
- The techniques of Korean wrestling (*ssireum*)
- Since the late 1990s, Mongolian grappling (the greatest influence)

Moves such as leg picks and rear throws out of the ring could not be explained by traditional kimarite. In response, the sumo elders studied the ancient records searching for new techniques to add to the kimarite list. In 2001, twelve new kimarite were added to make a total of eighty-two kimarite. Some of the new kimarite include rear lift out (*okuritsuridashi*) and underarm-forward body drop (*tsutaezori*), which is performed by ducking under the opponent's armpit. Stablemaster Oyama, a walking encyclopedia of sumo, said, "Kimarite is part of sumo culture. We think of them as our treasure."[11]

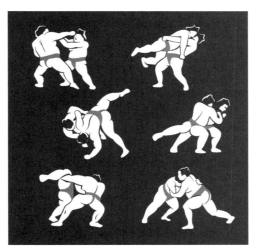

Sumo techniques.
(Photo © Sahua, Dreamstime.)

Overview Conclusion

In this chapter, we saw that there are solid arguments for thinking sumo is the root of jujitsu. We also considered some well-known martial artists who include sumo in their martial arts training. Then we introduced the history and practice of sumo, and finally we looked at the evolution of sumo's winning moves (kimarite). The chapter "Sumo Wrestling Case Studies" will uncover the techniques and tactics of sumo in depth; "Sumo and MMA" will expose the technical connections sumo has within MMA; and the final chapter will illustrate sumo's winning moves from an MMA perspective in detailed photos.

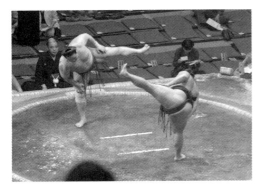

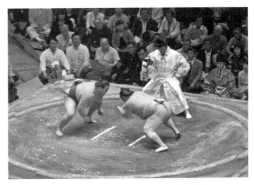

Two sumo wrestlers are performing *shiko*, which is executed ritually to drive away bad spirits from the dohyo before each bout. Shiko, foot stomping, is a signature sumo exercise where each leg is lifted as straight and as high as possible to the side while maintaining good posture, and then brought down to stomp on the ground with tremendous force. In training at the sumostable, shiko may be repeated hundreds of times in a row. This is amazing conditioning, especially because the rikishi are greatly known for their monstrous power and explosiveness, not their flexibility.

(Photo courtesy of Yves Picq, Wikimedia Commons.)

Two sumo wrestlers making the initial charge (*tachi-ai*) at each other at the beginning of a match. The initial collision of two rikishi can generate an incredible one ton or more of force.

(Photo courtesy of Gusjer, Flikr.)

Chapter 2

Sumo Wrestling Case Studies

Introduction

In this chapter, we will study a specially selected group of professional rikishi for their wrestling style. As you will see, some wrestlers' body types and fighting styles can vary dramatically, and their bouts can be quite interesting when they get together in the ring. When it comes to fighting styles in sumo, there are basically two types: traditional belt-grabbing sumo wrestling and pushing sumo wrestling. Undoubtedly, there are many rikishi who are proficient in both styles of sumo wrestling, but usually a rikishi focuses on either a pushing style or a belt-grabbing style. Techniques and tactics are presented in detail so readers might add some of these sumo moves to their own martial arts repertoire.

Case Study 1: Mainoumi—"Department Store of Techniques"

In sumo, size certainly matters, but technique matters as well. A case study in size versus technique naturally leads to the popular Japanese rikishi Mainoumi. He was five feet seven and a half inches in height and only 220 pounds, a very small person by sumo standards. Mainoumi used up to thirty-three kinds of kimarite in his wrestling days. Because of his broad use of kimarite, he was nicknamed "Department Store of Techniques" (Waza no Depaato). Mainoumi has said, "The eighty-two kimarite enhance the value of sumo."[12] Mainoumi rose to the *komusubi* rank, the fourth level from the top, an incredible achievement for a small rikishi in a field of giants.

Mainoumi was one of the most popular rikishi in the 1990s as his great fighting spirit and broad use of kimarite made him stand apart from the other much larger rikishi he was wrestling. For a smaller rikishi, Mainoumi's strong judo background combined with his remarkable physical strength and agility made him a very formidable opponent. It was not uncommon for Mainoumi to win against rikishi who outweighed him by two to almost three times. A solid push from a larger rikishi would launch him in the air. He would also lose if a larger rikishi achieved a dominating hold on him. Because of this, Mainoumi would at the start of the bout feint a forward charge and then quickly jump off the line of attack. Frequently, the larger rikishi's forward momentum was committed enough that he would fall to the ground. If that didn't work, Mainoumi was prepared to get beside or behind his opponent and push him out of the ring or down to the ground.

Opponents started to catch on to Mainoumi's tactics and wouldn't commit themselves to a full-on charge at the start of the bout. The match would be downgraded to a noncommitted pushing contest. This was a contest Mainoumi couldn't win, so he would slip or jump to his opponent's side or back. He had plenty of strength and leg techniques to throw opponents once he was in a dominant position. Mainoumi was most vulnerable when squared up in front of his opponent. This occurred often when facing other smaller, fast rikishi like him.

Mainoumi, at the initial charge, would commonly employ quick and cunning moves, shocking both the opponent and the audience. For instance, he would use an unconventional sumo wrestling technique called "deceiving the cat" (*nekodamashi*). At the start of the bout, a rikishi abruptly claps his hands together just in front of his opponent's face without touching it. The objective of this technique is to cause the opponent to close his eyes for a moment and distract him briefly, giving an advantage to the hand-clapping rikishi. This technique can be risky as, if it fails, it exposes the rikishi to his opponent's onslaught. The hand clapping is not that difficult. The hard part is how the opponent's brief distraction is instantly leveraged to gain the advantage. However, this trick will probably work only once on a particular opponent, as he will be expecting it the next time.

The *mawashi* is the belt worn by the rikishi. "The law of the ring" is that the one who dominates his opponent's mawashi with a controlling grip will almost certainly win the match. Mainoumi considered his opponent's mawashi his "lifeline": if he did not grip it, he would lose. Mainoumi has said that where you grab the mawashi determines how you can turn or throw your opponent. The mawashi grip gives the rikishi the greatest leverage.

According to Mainoumi, "The worst scenario for a small rikishi is having to face a strong head-on charge. If this happens he will be overpowered and pushed out instantly. This is the most dangerous thing. To absorb the bigger rikishi thrusting, he can pull back his shoulder quickly and weaken the power of the attack. You have to be innovative. Respond flexibly in order to cope with a bigger foe."[13] To be innovative and flexible, the martial artist must dig deep into his technical repertoire to unearth appropriate solutions to the problems presented.

A prime example of Mainoumi's advice can be seen in the November 1991 match he had with Akebono (Chad George Haheo Rowan). At more than five hundred pounds,

Akebono was over twice Mainoumi's weight and, at six feet eight inches, he was much taller. Mainoumi won the match by using a kimarite that had not been used in twenty years in a major tournament, a move judged by most observers to be a triple-attack force out (*mitokorozeme*) but that was officially judged an inside leg trip (*uchigake*). They are both leg techniques, which Mainoumi prefers, as they are an effective way for small rikishi to take down massive opponents.

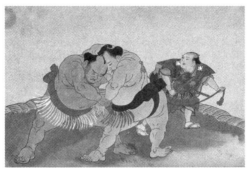

Two sumo wrestlers with a referee. Color woodcut. Nineteenth century.
(Photo courtesy of Fae, Wikimedia Commons.)

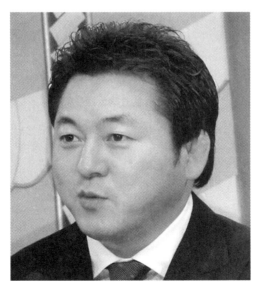

Sumo wrestler Mainoumi.
(Photo courtesy of FourTildes, Wikimedia Commons.)

Case Study 2: Akebono—Grand Champion, Yokozuna

Akebono, a Hawaiian, was a very formidable opponent. In 1993 he became the first foreign-born rikishi promoted to *yokozuna*, the highest rank in sumo. Akebono was a powerful and longtime yokozuna. His reign in that rank lasted almost eight years. He used all of his incredible physical attributes to his advantage. His very strong and long arms were merciless when pushing or thrusting into an opponent, sometimes knocking rikishi out of the ring with just one or two movements. Akebono could practically not be beat if his opponent failed to secure a grip on his mawashi. Also, his balance was excellent compared to many other very large rikishi. Akebono said, "They [a lot of people] don't realize how much hard work, learning and determination you got to put in. Not even Michael Jordan was great right away."[14]

Akebono told *National Geographic*, "People see these big fat guys tossing each other around the ring, and it's hard to understand that this is a mental sport. But the mental side, the spiritual side, is a lot more important than the body. If you can't get yourself in the right frame of mind intellectually, you can't win."[15]

> *Strength alone is not enough to make a grand champion. In sumo there are three ideals: spirit, skill and body. You cannot be chosen to be a Yokozuna unless you have these qualities. So you must be a great human being as well as a great wrestler.*
> —Wakamatsu Oyakata, sumo coach and elder[16]

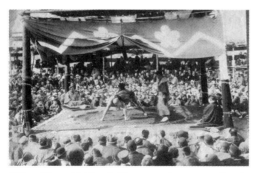

"Wrestling at Tokyo": Two wrestlers engaging in a match of sumo in a ring at Tokyo, with referees standing and sitting nearby and a large crowd of Japanese in Western-style clothing watching. Hand-colored albumen photograph by unknown photographer, 1890s.

(Photo courtesy of Kükator, Wikimedia Commons.)

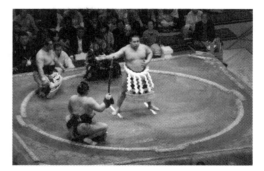

Yokozuna Kakuryu performing the *yokozuna dohyo-iri*, grand champion ring-entering ceremony, on day eleven of the 2014 May Grand Sumo Tournament in Tokyo, Japan. Date: May 21, 2014.

(Photo courtesy of Simon Q, Flikr.)

Case Study 3: Konishiki—Ozeki "Meat Bomb"

Konishiki is the first foreign-born rikishi to be promoted to *ozeki*, the second highest rank in sumo. Konishiki (Saleva'a Fuauli Atisano'e) is a Hawaiian like Akebono. Also, Konishiki was the heaviest rikishi ever in sumo history, at six feet one and a half inches and 630 pounds at career maximum weight. Because of his great weight the Japanese affectionately nicknamed him "Meat Bomb." Konishiki was very close to the promotion to yokozuna, but unfortunately he never made it. The popular Hawaiian rikishi, Akebono and Konishiki, helped make sumo better known around the world.

Because Konishiki lacked technique compared to the other more experienced rikishi, he had to compensate by using his weight and power. Konishiki has said his sumo fighting style was "strictly offensive."[17] He did not try to counter his opponent's moves defensively. By applying his monstrous size and strength, Konishiki just tried offensively to force his opponent out of the ring. His tactics worked so well they helped him achieve the much esteemed ozeki rank, the rank right before yokozuna. Although these offensive tactics usually only work for the larger rikishi, it is important to see how the larger rikishi wrestles, as this will help to show how the smaller rikishi devise ways to counter them.

Here Konishiki describes his sumo fighting style in depth: "My style is just using hands more. It's like a boxing style, with just heavy punching. Just learning how to move my hands."[18] "My style is all power. Hitting and just powering people out. Using my hands like a football pass blocker that is my style of wrestling and I guess that is my strongest point. If I can hit a guy in the jaw and get him off balance. . . . Either you're going to take a blow or I'm going to take a blow, but I'm not taking any. I'm the one who wants to give the blows. I'm trying to learn how to counter things that I'm not too good at, because when people grab my belt I have trouble. The smaller people because of the technique and because the ways that their style is different. It is like opposite of what I do."[19] It is interesting to note that Konishiki states that pushing sumo and belt-grabbing sumo are rather opposite styles. The pushing sumo style relies on physical attributes such as weight, power, and speed, while the belt-grabbing or clinching style is more of a learned technical skill.

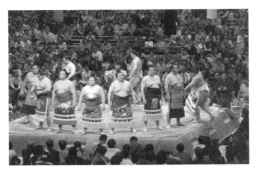

Professional sumo wrestlers perform the ring-entering ceremony (*dohyo-iri*). May 2005.

(Photo courtesy of Yves Picq, Wikimedia Commons.)

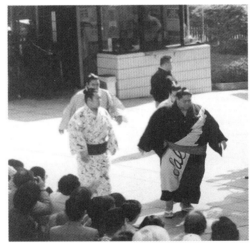

Sumo wrestler Konishiki and entourage, Ryogoku, Tokyo. May 1996.

(Photo courtesy of Howcheng, Wikimedia Commons.)

Case Study 4: Terao—"Iron Man" of Sumo

Terao was a slender, popular Japanese rikishi who had a unique sumo career. Terao was six feet one inch tall and 260 pounds, a little bigger than some smaller rikishi but definitely much smaller than most. He had a long family history of rikishi. Also Terao had the distinction of having an extraordinary long professional sumo career, lasting twenty-three years from 1979 until 2002, even though he was a smaller rikishi. Because of this Terao was nicknamed the "Iron Man" (*Tetsujin*) of sumo.

Terao was a smaller rikishi but with a very different wrestling style than Mainoumi. Terao was known to be fast and agile in the ring, and he used pushing and thrusting techniques on his opponent. His pushing sumo style worked best when his opponent stayed away from his belt. Because of his small size compared to the bigger rikishi, he was at a disadvantage, but with his fast movement and continuous thrusts to the body, he won many matches. Terao's wrestling style many times involved *tsuppari*, a fury of short pushes to the opponent's face and upper torso using alternating flailing open-handed pushes like a windmill, and then releasing the pressure suddenly and quickly executing the common kimarite *hatakikomi*, which is a slap down that sends the opponent crashing forward onto the dohyo. Terao even beat the immense Konishiki with this tactic.

Recall what Mainoumi said about the small rikishi facing a strong head-on charge.[20] He would be overpowered and lose almost immediately. If Terao could not get out of the way, he was susceptible to being overpowered and pushed out. You could say Terao's fighting style was an interesting combination of Akebono or Konishiki and Mainoumi: getting off the line of attack like Mainoumi and merciless thrusting like the bigger rikishi. With his remarkable long career, Terao's highest rank was *sekiwake*, the third highest rank in professional sumo wrestling.

Case Study 5: Open-Hand Attacks

Martial artists could benefit from studying the sumo way of open-hand pushes, slaps, and thrusts. Closed-fist attacks are illegal in sumo, so rikishi have become very proficient in open-hand attacks. As described earlier, very successful rikishi such as Akebono, Konishiki, and Terao relied mostly on the open-hand attack style of sumo to win their matches. Don Wilson, the kickboxing champion and actor, once mentioned that open-hand attacks are safer to perform, as fist attacks have a high likelihood of breaking your hand. Wilson confirmed this by his observations as a commenter at a very early Ultimate Fighting Championship (UFC), when fighters didn't wear gloves, and most of them injured their hands while fighting with their fists. Gloves are primarily used not to protect the person being hit, but to prevent to striker's fist from breaking.

How do rikishi condition themselves for open-hand attacks? One major way is by using the *teppo*, which is a wooden pillar approximately the diameter of a telephone pole. Teppo trains one to block an oncoming opponent. By continuously slapping the teppo, rikishi toughen and strengthen their hands. The rikishi also slap and push against the teppo while sliding their feet back and forth in unison with their hands to put their weight behind the movements. This improves their balance, coordination, and rhythm, also strengthening the muscles of the legs, hips, and arms. Teppo training could be seen as similar to karate's padded striking-post training (*makiwara*). Gichin Funakoshi said that as he was spreading karate throughout Japan, "Several gigantic sumo champions also sought instruction (although punching and kicking were not allowed in sumo, open-hand attacks were, and the wrestlers wanted to learn how to make more effective thrusts). . . ."[21]

Rikishi sliding their feet in unison with their hand movements creates a very powerful dynamic. The way rikishi move across the ring could benefit other martial artists. They move by sliding their feet so they have better balance. Also, when they are sliding their feet, the pad of the big toe never leaves the ground. Rikishi focus their weight on the insides of their feet. The big toe plays a major role in balance.[22] Try to balance on your two feet on your heels as compared to balancing on your big toe area, and you will see how critical the big toe is in your balancing ability. Without proper balance, your open-hand attacks and grappling takedowns would be much less effective. Moreover, if you have poor balance, you can be taken down more easily.

There is another part of the body of importance to the rikishi. When the rikishi is performing any movements (open-hand attacks or grappling takedowns) that utilize the hand, the end point for their energy release is the palm area of their pinky finger side. Just as the natural form and function of the big toe give them better balance, by focusing their energy into the pinky finger side of their palm, they create the greatest conductor of force into their opponent. When thrusting, rikishi keep their wrists between their elbows for the best leverage. They use the pinky side of their palm when thrusting, not their fingers. The hand and arm make it so effective because the natural motion of pushing your hand forward causes the pinky finger side of the palm, which is quite solid, to lead and make first contact. Simply by using their feet and hands in unison, they can dramatically improve their balance and optimize the projection of energy into their opponent.[23]

Some of sumo's open-hand attacks can be particularly brutal. One of these devastating open-hand attacks is a thrust or push to your opponent's throat (*nodowa*). This thrust or push is performed with the opponent's throat falling in between your thumb and four fingers. This technique is not strangling by gripping the throat, an illegal move in sumo. Instead, it is a technique to push your opponent's center of gravity upward and backward by only thrusting or pushing on the throat.[24] The other devastating open-hand attack is a head slap (*harite*). It is a common technique in professional sumo used to stun your opponent so you can obtain a dominant grip on his belt (mawashi). This head slap can be quite disorienting to your opponent and can be delivered with such force as to possibly knock him out.[25] Even though open-hand thrusts, pushes, and slaps may not have the stopping power of a closed fist, the safety factor of not breaking your hand as easily as with fist strikes is a definite advantage.

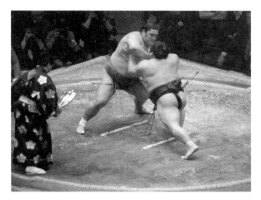

Okinoumi (left) vs. Takekaze (right) at the 2014 January Grand Sumo Tournament in Tokyo.

(Courtesy of Gregg Tavares, Wikimedia Commons.)

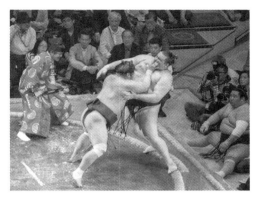

Sumo wrestlers fighting: one pushing the other in the face. Myogiryu (left) vs. Gagamaru at the 2014 May Grand Sumo Tournament in Tokyo, Japan. The open-hand attacks in sumo may not have the stopping power of a closed fist, but they offer the advantage of not breaking your hand as easily.

(Photo courtesy Simon Q, Flickr.)

Case Study 6: Dominating Techniques

Aggressiveness by driving forward is a critical principle of sumo. In many of sumo's historic bouts, a rikishi's forward charge has been decisive in attaining victory. Kisenosato, a successful rikishi, said, "My ideal style is making a strong charge, keeping the momentum, forcing out the opponent straight away, I always aim to do this."[26] Stablemaster Naruto (Takanosato) instructs his rikishi Kisenosato, "Techniques evolve naturally if you move forward. So I always tell him to move forward."[27] Moving forward puts your opponent on the defensive, so you can capitalize on his reactions. The best defense is a good offense.

Stablemaster Naruto says focus on sumo basics, which include understanding the angle of the initial charge and keeping the arms tightly against the sides. If rikishi practice the basics thoroughly, they can apply them to more advanced techniques. This concept of keeping the arms tightly against the sides or closing the armpits is a common theme in Japanese martial arts. According to the *Kodokan New Japanese-English Dictionary of Judo, waki wo shimeru* (to close the armpits) means, "To lower the arms to minimize or eliminate the space between the body and the arms," which is "a basic and important technical point in judo and in Japanese martial arts in general."[28]

Keeping the arms tightly against the sides gives you better mechanical advantage for defensive and offensive techniques. For instance, having the arms tightly against the sides helps the rikishi keep his opponent from gaining inside control and makes getting inside control easier. The double-underhooks clinch (*ryo-shitate*) is a powerful inside control technique that commonly leads to victory in a sumo match. Also, the rikishi who has his hands on the inside is better able to shoot under for a leg attack. For instance, the kimarite leg pick (*ashitori*) and ankle pick (*susotori*) are shooting under-leg attacks, which are made much more effective by gaining inside control first before shooting under. Rikishi are always struggling for inside control, as inside control gives the rikishi some of the best leverage to dominate his opponent.

As just shown earlier, the double-underhooks clinch is often used to prevail in a sumo match. However, there is a popular sumo counter to this clinch, namely the *kannuki* hold. The kannuki hold is performed by wrapping both arms around the outside of the opponent's arms that are gripping you in the double-underhooks clinch. You lift him up by the armpits, removing his leverage and making his arms practically useless. Taller rikishi are better at this defense, as it is easier for them to lift up their opponent. This defensive hold often causes injuries to the elbows of the rikishi applying the double-underhooks clinch. Kannuki means "bolt" or "latch," like to a door. The armbar force down (*kimetaoshi*) is one kimarite that utilizes the kannuki hold. See the photos for armbar force down in chapter 4 for more details on this technique.

One essential tactic successful rikishi must keep in mind when performing most kimarite is balance breaking (*kuzushi*). Balance breaking is any maneuver used to unbalance your opponent just before attempting to take him down. It is usually performed while trying to maintain your own balance. Balance breaking the opponent before taking him down dramatically decreases the amount of energy needed to complete the takedown. This is especially important when smaller rikishi take down larger rikishi. One relatively easy way to unbalance the opponent is to go with his movements. For instance, if he pushes you, you pull, and if he pulls you, you push. Mainoumi alludes to this idea of going with the flow when he says, "To absorb the bigger rikishi thrusting he can pull back his shoulder quickly and weaken the power of the attack."[29] This going with the flow, which could easily unbalance his opponent, must have set up many opportunities for Mainoumi to employ his vast array of kimarite.

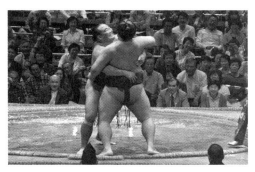

A sumo wrestler battles for the double-underhooks clinch (ryo-shitate). October 1, 2012.

(Photo courtesy of 江戸村のとくぞう, "Tokuzou of Edo Village," Wikimedia Commons.)

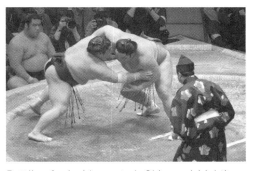

Battling for inside control. Okinoumi (right) vs. Takekaze (left) at the 2014 January Grand Sumo Tournament in Tokyo. January 25, 2014.

(Photo courtesy of Gregg Tavares, Wikimedia Commons.)

Case Studies Conclusion

As you can gather from the sumo case studies, large rikishi who have strong head-on charges tend to win. As mentioned earlier, many of sumo's historic bouts were won by a strong head-on charge. We could have discussed many other colorful and successful rikishi, but the few chosen here exemplify the styles of sumo wrestling very well. To paraphrase Mainoumi, rikishi today rely on sheer brute strength and should practice more kimarite; in fifty or one hundred years, unused kimarite will be forgotten and thought of as myth. He says it is not too late to do something about it. Of the eighty-two kimarite, some have never been used in Grand Sumo Tournaments. Mainoumi didn't even perform them in his bouts. As more rikishi from diverse backgrounds work their way up the sumo ranks, the winning moves and tactics will continue to evolve.

Chapter 3

Sumo and MMA

Introduction

We turn now to mixed martial arts (MMA), which offers more tools for achieving victory than sumo and is a very different combat sport. Of course, size and strength matter a lot in MMA contests, but with the rules allowing more highly effective strikes, positions, and submissions, the bout contains many more fight equalizers than the David and Goliath sumo match. Some rikishi have competed in MMA with limited success. Rikishi have difficultly adapting to MMA, as their lack of speed compared to a skilled smaller foe and their large frames make them especially vulnerable to strikes and submissions.

The free-movement phase, when both combatants are standing and there is no gripping between them, is addressed somewhat in sumo with open-handed thrusts, slaps, and pushes. These open-handed techniques are not designed for a knockout but to move the rikishi out of the sumo ring. In MMA these open-handed moves would be less effective, because knocking an opponent out of a cage or even a boxing ring is much more difficult and is not the objective in that sport. Plus, the dynamics of takedowns and strikes are much different against an MMA cage wall than an open sumo ring.

Ground fighting is not dealt with in sumo at all, because in a sumo match, once a rikishi touches anything on the ground beyond the soles of his feet, the match is over. Submissions, a requirement for success in MMA competitions, are not really taught in sumo. The only submission-type kimarite are armlock-like throws against the elbow. Some examples are the popular armlock throw (*kotenage*), the rarely used armbar throw (*tottari*), and the very rarely used armbar-throw counter (*sakatottari*). Plus, several major sumo moves require the use of a belt to grip the opponent. In MMA competitions there is usually no belt to grip, but in gi-wearing contests, a belt is available for use as well as in many self-defense situations. It is therefore apparent that the means of achieving victory in an MMA competition and in a sumo match are vastly different.

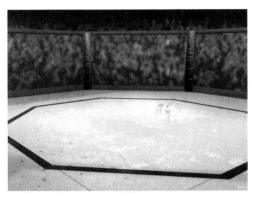

Mixed martial arts fighting arena.
(Photo courtesy of Neil Lockhart, Shutterstock.)

The Clinch Phase

But there are significant similarities between these two combat sports. Mostly, sumo techniques deal with the standing clinch phase of hand-to-hand fighting. The clinch, yori, is when there is some sort of gripping between the combatants while they are standing. There are numerous types of clinches. The standing clinch is one of the three major phases of hand-to-hand fighting and MMA. Combatants usually clinch when one of them is defending a takedown or as they strike each other. It may not be as well known as the free-movement phase (standing strikes with no grips) and the ground phase, but it is just as critical.

In an unarmed single fight, the most powerful clinches provide you with the most control of your opponent's movements. Solid grips on your opponent's head or torso offer this valuable control. A powerful clinch ties up your opponent and takes much of his striking ability away. On the other hand, a simple wrist grab does not control your opponent's movements much and as such is a poor clinch.

A good standing clinch can stop much of your opponent's striking ability, and it gives you many options: striking from the clinch, standing submissions, takedowns to ground fighting, or disengaging to the free-movement phase to strike. Depending on the dominance of your standing clinch, your opponent has those options as well. The clinch is like a hinge that connects the other two phases of combat. Being proficient in the clinch gives you the ability to dictate where the fight will lead—to the free-movement phase or to the ground phase. As shown in professional boxing and MMA competitions around the globe, avoiding the clinch is very difficult, even when facing a lesser adversary. That is why clinching skills are so important.

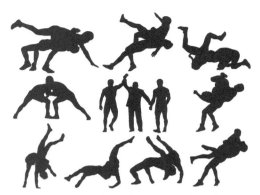

Clinches and takedowns are a vital part of the fight game, but they are often overlooked. (Photo courtesy of only4denn, Can Stock Photo.)

The Over-Under Clinch

Interestingly enough, the over-under clinch that is very popular in sumo is the most used type of clinch in MMA contests. If you look at the illustrations that describe the eighty-two sumo kimarite listed by the Japan Sumo Association, you will notice that the over-under clinch is extremely prevalent. Renzo Gracie and John Danaher state that "the over-under clinch is undoubtedly the most common form of clinch in MMA competition."[30] This use of the over-under clinch is a common thread between sumo and MMA. For both combat sports, one major goal of this clinch is to take your opponent to the ground.

As its name implies, the over-under clinch (see photo on next page) is where both combatants have one overhook and one underhook. The overhook or overarm, *uwate*, is performed by placing an arm over the opponent's arm and securing it. The underhook or underarm, *shitate*, secures the opponent's upper body with your arm placed under the opponent's arm. The underhook is the offensive position, while the overhook is the defensive and weaker hold. When in the over-under clinch, your head is usually on the side of your overhooked arm, as this puts weight on your opponent's underhooked arm, which nullifies some of his powerful control with the underhook. With this clinch a combatant should have his shoulder (underhook side) buried into the opponent's chest, pushing in. For better balance, you are usually in a staggered stance with your lead leg on the side you are underhooking your opponent.

The positions of the combatants when they are in the over-under clinch mirror one another, thus creating a neutral position. This neutral position is created as each combatant has an equal opportunity to attack and defend. Even though the over-under clinch is a neutral position, it still greatly controls your opponent's torso and is therefore a powerful clinch. In this clinch, technical skill and physical attributes, such as size and strength, play important roles in determining the advantage.

Why is the over-under clinch the most commonly used clinch in sumo and MMA? One reason is that it is a powerful neutral clinch, so it is easier to attain than a powerful dominant clinch such as the double-underhooks clinch. Most importantly, the over-under clinch, for a neutral clinch, controls the opponent's striking arms the best. The collar-and-elbow clinch is also a powerful neutral clinch, but it does not control the opponent's striking arms that well. In some other grappling sports, like folkstyle and Greco-Roman wrestling, strikes are forbidden; therefore, the collar-and-elbow clinch is much more commonly used. In sumo and MMA, head and body strikes are always a threat in the clinch. Both of these combat sports have evolved a preference for the over-under clinch because of the crucial need to protect from the devastating strikes of the opponent's arms. Also, part of the reason rikishi use the over-under clinch so often is because it gives them a grip closest to their opponent's belt. This gives the rikishi maximum gripping control over his opponent. Because the over-under clinch is an easy-to-attain neutral clinch that gives the best striking protection for a neutral clinch, this clinch provides an important link between sumo and MMA. As you can gather from the illustrations in this book, sumo has many answers to the riddle of the over-under clinch—answers that send the opponent crashing to the ground.

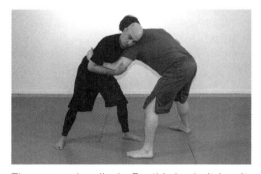

The over-under clinch. For this book, it is critical to understand the over-under clinch, as most of the technical photos start from this position. The over-under clinch is the most commonly used clinch in both sumo and MMA. (Photo by Kristopher Schoenleber.)

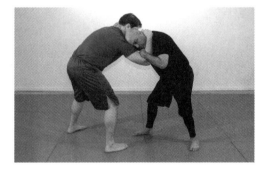

The collar-and-elbow clinch. The collar-and-elbow clinch is also a powerful neutral clinch like the over-under clinch, but it does not control the opponent's striking arms as well as the over-under clinch. This makes the over-under clinch a much better choice for sumo and MMA, where strikes are allowed. In some other grappling sports, like folkstyle and Greco-Roman wrestling, strikes are forbidden; therefore, the collar-and-elbow clinch is much more commonly used. (Photo by Kristopher Schoenleber.)

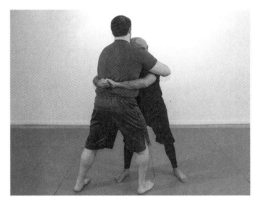

The double-underhooks clinch. This dominant clinch is usually attained after locking up in the over-under clinch.

(Photo by Kristopher Schoenleber.)

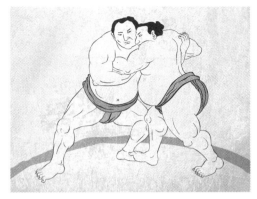

Japanese sumo wrestlers in the over-under clinch. Illustration done in Japanese wood block print style.

(Photo courtesy of patrimonio, Can Stock Photo.)

Why the Takedown?

After the opponent hits the ground from a takedown, the ground phase begins. In the ground phase the combatants can employ strikes or submissions from a variety of ground positions, which gives them the best control over their opponent's movements. Therefore, for many MMA fighters this is their preferred phase of combat, as discussed in more detail below. Performing a successful takedown on your opponent gives you a much greater opportunity to achieve a dominant top position on the ground. This takedown to a dominant top position when first entering the ground phase is much more effective than pulling your opponent into your guard and ground fighting from a bottom position. The guard is where you are on your back or buttocks with your legs in front of your opponent. If used properly, the bottom guard can be a powerful position for performing many offensive and defensive techniques, but a dominant top position on the ground is always preferred by submission grapplers.

From your dominant top position, your opponent not only has to carry your weight, but your movements, submissions, and strikes are also much better as gravity is on your side and you have a lot more variations of techniques available to you. Renzo Gracie and John Danaher said it nicely: "In a ground fight, it is always desirable to be on top, in the most controlling position possible. If, however, you find yourself in the bottom position, the guard is the best place to be."[31] Because practically all fights start standing, it makes sense that strong takedowns are one of the best ways to enter the ground phase and immediately achieve a controlling top position.

Why is the ground phase preferred by many MMA fighters? Why should an MMA fighter be skillful in taking the fight to the ground with takedowns? The ground phase is preferred by many MMA fighters for a number of reasons. Real dominance in an unarmed single fight is generally achieved by superior body contact (controlling the opponent's body), which can be used to negate your opponent's striking and submission ability. The free-movement phase gives the fighter no grips and therefore no body contact. The standing clinch gives the fighter some body contact. Finally, the ground phase gives the fighter the most possibilities for superior body contact to dominate his opponent with strikes and submissions.

Size and strength are not as threatening to a skilled ground fighting specialist as they might be to other fighters because the ground phase is a learned skill that nullifies many of your opponent's physical attributes. Additionally, some MMA fighters are not well versed in the ground phase, so it would be beneficial for the ground specialist to take the opponent out of his element. In both MMA fights and street fights, moreover, there is a high likelihood that the fight will end up on the ground anyway, either as the result of a fall during the struggle or by design from a determined takedown. So being well versed in the ground phase is a way of being very prepared for the inevitable. Effective take-downs help you get to the ground phase more safely and quickly so you do not receive as much punishment from strikes in the free-movement phase and the clinch phase.

Detailed ground fighting is beyond the scope of this book, especially because sumo wrestling is not a ground-fighting martial art. Nevertheless, the benefits of taking the fight to the ground had to be discussed as most of sumo's techniques are takedowns, and it would be reasonable to know why you would want to go to the ground in a fight. There are countless quality ground-fighting instructional books and videos on the market today that can help educate you in the ground phase of combat.

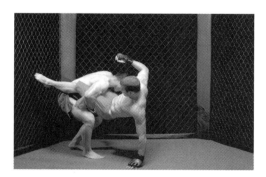

MMA fighter taking down his opponent in the cage.
(Photo courtesy of nickp37, Can Stock Photo.)

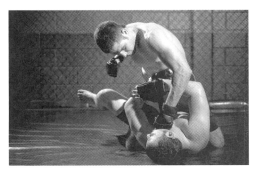

The ground-fighting phase is preferred by many MMA fighters for a number of reasons. Real dominance in an unarmed single fight is generally achieved by superior body contact (controlling the opponent's body), which can be used to negate your opponent's striking and submission ability. The free-movement phase gives the fighter no grips and therefore no body contact. The standing clinch gives the fighter some body contact. Finally, the ground phase gives the fighter the most possibilities for superior body contact to dominate his opponent with strikes and submissions.

(Photo courtesy of Antonio Diaz, Can Stock Photo.)

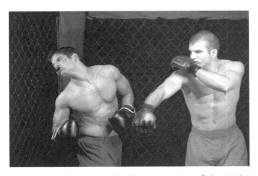

Effective takedowns help you get to the ground phase more safely and quickly so you do not receive as much punishment from strikes in the free-movement phase and the clinch phase.

(Photo courtesy of nickp37, Can Stock Photo.)

The Complete MMA Fighter

Sumo can improve your clinch, which includes performing takedowns and the defenses against them. Understandably, the clinch phase is just one part of the larger fight game. Clinching skills alone are not enough to succeed consistently in today's MMA competitions. Cross-training is needed to be skillful in all the phases of hand-to-hand fighting, and a little sumo may help balance out the equation. Some sumo techniques could be helpful in MMA to enhance an already-solid base of striking and ground fighting.

To truly understand the need for cross-training, one just has to look at UFC 1: The Beginning in November 1993. Single-style martial artists fought each other: for instance, a kickboxer (Gerard Gordeau) versus a sumo wrestler (Teila Tuli) and a BJJ practitioner (Royce Gracie) versus a Western boxer (Art Jimmerson). One might be quick to dismiss sumo as ineffective because the kickboxer finished the fight quickly with strong striking. But if you look at the fight between the BJJ practitioner and the Western boxer, the BJJ practitioner finished the fight just as easily as the kickboxer. Would you now say Western boxing is ineffective in MMA? Most MMA fighters today incorporate some form of boxing into their game. Having boxing or sumo skills alone is a recipe for disaster in modern MMA competition. Today with the use of gloves, rounds, time limits, and other rules in modern MMA competition, even the BJJ practitioner isn't guaranteed a victory. To be a competitive MMA fighter today, you must be a complete fighter, having familiarity with all the phases of fighting.

Today's MMA uses four major martial arts: muay Thai, Western boxing, BJJ, and Western wrestling (folkstyle, freestyle, and Greco-Roman). Of course, there are many other martial arts used in MMA, but the abovementioned are the four major ones. Each adds to the MMA fighter's arsenal. Muay Thai and Western boxing cover the free-movement phase and clinch phase for striking, while BJJ covers the ground phase mostly with submissions and, somewhat, with the clinch for takedowns. Finally, Western wrestling in all its variations covers the clinch phase with takedowns and the ground phase with positional balance on top. Sumo wrestling would fit into this mix of the four major martial arts as an Asian form of wrestling with its clinching and takedown skills and to a lesser extent the free-movement phase with its open-handed thrusts, pushes, and slaps.

Three basic fighting styles have emerged in modern MMA. Most successful MMA fighters are well versed in at least one of these three styles. After the style is described, the reason why sumo wrestling skills can benefit that particular MMA style will be discussed.

- "Sprawl and brawl" fighters are strikers who prefer to be in the free-movement phase and brawl (strike) it out for the knockout. In this strategy, the fighter realizes the danger of the clinch and takedown to the ground phase. Hence, the fighter has learned to sprawl to avoid takedowns and knows just enough ground fighting to survive to get to his feet and look for the knockout. Sumo skills could benefit "sprawl and brawl" fighters because they absolutely need as much takedown defense as they can get, and sumo clinches, takedowns, and their defenses will give them an advantage. As will be examined more in depth shortly, Lyoto "The Dragon" Machida is primarily a "sprawl and brawl" fighter who uses sumo takedowns and their defenses brilliantly in MMA competition.

- Submission grapplers are MMA fighters who prefer to take the fight to the ground where they can gain positional dominance and work for the submission. This type of fighter exploits the many advantages of ground fighting we discussed earlier. However, a major weakness of many submission grapplers is their clinching and takedown ability. Sumo wrestling has many no-gi-cloth-required takedowns from the clinch that could clearly benefit the submission grappler. As discussed earlier, effective takedowns are a much better option than pulling guard and fighting from the bottom.

- "Ground and pound" fighters tend to be big, strong Western wrestlers who like to clinch, takedown their opponent to the ground, and pound (strike) their way to victory from any top position. Understandably, this type of fighter already has excellent clinching and takedown ability, but because this ability is so critical to their success, looking at sumo clinches and takedowns would not be a bad idea as they could definitely learn something of value. Sumo has many variations of takedowns probably not known by most grapplers that would fit nicely into the "ground and pound" fighter's repertoire.

Additionally, many folkstyle and freestyle wrestling takedowns (single and double legs) attack the lower body, requiring that your lower legs (instep, shin, or knee) slide on the ground to penetrate your opponent's defenses from a changed lower level. From a self-defense standpoint, if you rely on these types of takedowns when not on a padded surface, like on the street, your legs will most likely be injured. Sumo takedowns are much safer in that respect as the takedowns have evolved in accordance with the rules of sumo. The rikishi would lose the match if he slid his legs on the ground for a takedown because only the soles of the feet can touch the ground in the sumo ring.

Especially because there are now weight divisions in most of modern MMA, the sumo diet and weight gain methods would be impractical for most. The sumo physique is also not practical for MMA, even in open-weight events, as great mobility is required to escape striking and submission attempts. But even though not all elements of sumo are usable in MMA, there are significant techniques and tactics that are very applicable to the MMA fighter's game.

Mitsuyo "Count Trouble" Maeda: Father of Brazilian Jiu-Jitsu

Long ago, there was a mixed martial arts genius who, if not for sumo, may not have become the legend that he is. Mitsuyo "Count Trouble" Maeda (1878–1941), the judo master who introduced his art to the Gracie family, first studied sumo as a boy under the watchful eye of his father. The records of Maeda's early years are sparse, but it has been said that Maeda's father was a formidable amateur sumo wrestler and he trained Maeda relentlessly from an early age. Maeda proved to be a gifted student in sumo. He won many local matches. Maeda and his family most likely realized, however, that because of Maeda's small build, it would be very difficult for him to become the sumo champion of Japan.

Maeda had an extremely strong fighting spirit and wanted to be a professional fighter someday. Because sumo was not ideally suited for him, he decided to switch to jujitsu and judo where size was not as vital for success. Maeda entered the Kodokan Judo Institute in 1895 and became an exceptional judo expert. He traveled across the globe to fulfill his dream of becoming a professional fighter. "For the next three decades, Maeda (his stage name was Conde Koma, 'Count Trouble') fought thousands of battles against every manner of professional and amateur wrestler and boxer, other Japanese judo and jujutsu men, savate exponents, local toughs, and barroom brawlers in every kind of venue imaginable—tournaments, boxing rings, wrestling mats, theaters, music halls, circuses, and bars. Maeda crossed the globe fighting: the United States, the United Kingdom, Spain, Portugal, Belgium, France, Cuba, Mexico, and most important, South America."[32] Maeda is said to have lost only a handful of bouts in his three decades of fighting.

Because of his vast experience in fighting contests with many different types of fighters across the globe, Maeda found that he had to modify traditional judo to suit his needs as a professional fighter. He even added techniques and tactics to his repertoire from other martial arts that he picked up in his worldwide travels, but he kept judo and sumo as his foundational systems. When Maeda settled in Brazil, he passed on his incomparable hard-won fighting techniques and tactics to Carlos Gracie, who in turn helped to create Brazilian jiu-jitsu. Today, Brazilian jiu-jitsu has become a worldwide martial arts phenomenon, all from the fertile seeds planted by Maeda almost a century ago.

Considering this book's detailed focus on the clinch phase of fighting, it would be appropriate to explore Maeda's possible use of the clinch phase. As a youngster, because Maeda was a smaller sumo player, he most likely had a clinching style of sumo wrestling. Maeda probably used the clinch early on as a small sumo player to nullify the larger sumo player's pushing, thrusting, and slapping open-hand attacks. This clinch worked almost the same way in his legendary MMA matches. The clinch stopped much of his opponent's striking ability so he could take his opponent down to the ground phase, where he would finish the fight. Therefore, it is important to understand, as discussed earlier in this chapter, that the clinch is the hinge or in-between stage of the two other phases of combat: the free-movement phase and the ground phase. This makes the clinch vital for success in single unarmed combat. The Gracie family almost certainly learned the importance of the clinch from Maeda and incorporated it into their no-holds-barred fighting style, which eventually became modern MMA.

Even though the Kodokan frowned upon Maeda's MMA fighting exploits, the Kodokan recognized Maeda's accomplishments in spreading judo across the globe as they promoted Maeda to sixth dan in 1929 and seventh dan in 1941 after his death. Sometimes called the "toughest man who ever lived," he is said to have won more than two thousand professional fights in his career. Without a doubt, Maeda achieved his dream of becoming a champion professional fighter. The essence of his fighting techniques and tactics are immortalized in Brazilian jiu-jitsu. And sumo was his first and foundational martial art.

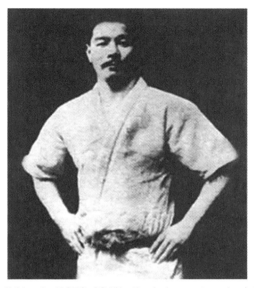

Mitsuyo "Count Trouble" Maeda (1878–1941), the judo master who introduced his art to the Gracie family, first studied sumo as a boy under the watchful eye of his father.
(Photo courtesy of EXECUTOR, Wikimedia Commons.)

Lyoto "The Dragon" Machida: Former UFC LHW Champion

A prime example of how an MMA fighter has incorporated sumo into his game is former UFC Light Heavyweight (LHW) Champion Lyoto "The Dragon" Machida. He has a strong sumo background, but his primary style is traditional Shotokan karate. Belém, Brazil, where Machida grew up, had a large Japanese colony. Machida learned sumo in this colony and began training and competing in sumo at twelve years of age.

Machida trained hard in sumo, even winning several sumo tournaments. Machida says in his book *Machida Karate-Do Mixed Martial Arts Techniques*, "I knew that every martial art had its strong points, and I figured the more martial arts I trained, the more weaknesses I would eliminate from my game."[33] His clinching, body-to-body sensitivity, balance breaking, and takedown skills were also vastly improved by his sumo experience.[34] In his book, Machida even demonstrates a sumo takedown from the over-under clinch that he found useful in MMA.[35] The sumo takedown looks to be a variation on the inner thigh sweep twist down (*uchimuso*).

Machida mentions that during his MMA fight with Rich Franklin in Japan in December 2003, his ability to keep his base—a skill he learned from sumo training—helped him achieve a top position on the ground after Franklin sunk in double underhooks for an attempted throw in the first round.[36] While in Franklin's guard, Machida escaped his triangle choke attempts and fired back with some solid punches. From a standing exchange of strikes, Machida knocked Franklin out unconscious in the second round. When Machida fought B. J. Penn in the K-1/Hero's 1 event in March 2005, he was able to keep the fight standing most of the time and control him in the clinch by using his evasive maneuvers and sumo training.[37] Machida won this tough MMA fight by unanimous decision. Also, Machida has successfully used the sumo kimarite outside leg trip (*sotogake*) numerous times in MMA competition. Outside leg trip is when your calf is wrapped around the opponent's calf from the outside so you can drive him down backward. (This outside leg trip is demonstrated in chapter 4 of this book.) During his MMA fight with Tito Ortiz in the UFC 84 event in May 2008, Machida stopped Ortiz's takedown attempts and took Ortiz down with ease using the outside leg trip. Machida beat Ortiz by unanimous decision.

In UFC 98 in May 2009, Machida faced Rashad Evans. With his stellar stand-up skills Machida KO'd Evans cold in the second round to win the UFC LHW title belt. When Machida fought UFC Hall of Famer Randy Couture in UFC 129 in April 2011, his takedown defense kept the fight standing long enough so he could knock Couture out with a surprising front kick in the second round. Machida's elusive standing style sometimes makes his opponents want to rush in to close the distance. The Bader vs. Machida fight showed why this is a big mistake. In UFC on Fox 4 in August 2012, Ryan Bader rushed Machida and ran into a right hand to the jaw that immediately knocked him out for Machida's win in the second round. When Machida faced Dan Henderson in UFC 157 in February 2013, Machida was able to mostly keep the fight on his feet even though Henderson is an expert Western wrestler. Machida even took Henderson down at the end of the first round with a trip. Machida won via split decision.

Machida is primarily an intelligent "sprawl and brawl" fighter. He grew up learning traditional Shotokan karate, and that is the strongest aspect of his game. Because karate is his main style, Machida prefers to stand and fight southpaw in a wide-angled Shotokan stance against his opponents. He uses high-level hit-and-run tactics with amazing footwork and powerful counterstriking. He has also extensively studied muay Thai, Western wrestling, judo, and sumo, which gives him the strong ability to attack in the clinch and thwart takedown attempts so he can stay on his feet. Machida has been pitted against some of the best takedown experts in modern MMA history—Couture and Henderson, for example—and has been able to keep the fight mostly standing and work his counterstriking magic. Also, with his black belt in BJJ, he is very dangerous in the ground phase if he ends up there. Most of his MMA wins via fight stoppage are from KOs/TKOs, and several are from ground submissions, although most of his fights in MMA are won via decision. With his diverse and comprehensive training background, he has a unique, powerful, unorthodox, and elusive MMA style.

Machida has achieved remarkable victories over some of the highest-level MMA fighters in the world. With his eclectic approach to martial arts training and very impressive MMA fight record, Machida has become one of the most formidable MMA fighters of his time. As we have noted, sumo is an important component of his MMA fighting game.

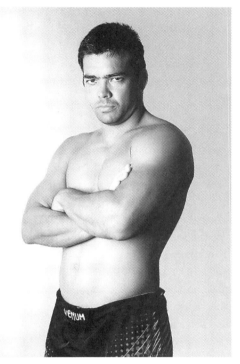

Lyoto Machida: A prime example of how an MMA fighter has incorporated sumo into his game is former UFC Light Heavyweight Champion Lyoto "The Dragon" Machida.
(Photo courtesy of Marcos Joel Reis, Wikimedia Commons.)

David vs. Goliath

In his very popular book *David and Goliath: Underdogs, Misfits, and the Art of Battling Giants,* Malcolm Gladwell explores the lessons behind the three-thousand-year-old biblical story of how the small, young David defeated the giant warrior Goliath. We can view the story from different angles and apply it to our own times. According to Gladwell, the David and Goliath metaphor for improbable victory is completely incorrect. When faced with an obstacle, are your strengths really strengths and weaknesses really weaknesses? The author demonstrates how we misinterpret the real meaning of advantage and disadvantage. From a combat perspective, a larger opponent's strengths can be his biggest weaknesses. Larger opponents tend to be less mobile and better targets for the smaller opponent to exploit. Too much of a "good thing" can be a weakness.

In Uyenishi's book *The Text-Book of Ju-Jutsu as Practiced in Japan,* the author describes jujitsu as the study of soft principles. Soft principles such as leverage and balance are the opposite of hard principles of strength and force.[38] From this description you can see that jujitsu is designed to help the weak defeat the strong. When jujitsu was first intro-duced to the West, its techniques were many times called tricks. The weaker jujitsu fighter essentially outsmarts his larger opponent—brains over brawn. The functionality of jujitsu is widely displayed in modern MMA competition, where takedowns, ground positions, and submissions are routinely used to defeat larger, stronger opponents. Sumo also applies these soft principles of leverage and balance to help small rikishi defeat much larger rikishi. By going back in time to the root of jujitsu, sumo, one can uncover gems that can be of much value to all martial artists.

Movement, balance, and leverage play a vital role in sumo takedowns. As shown in chapter 2, Mainoumi and Terao are smaller rikishi who have used their nimble move-ment to avoid the direct onslaught of much larger rikishi and to employ their own take-downs. Balance is crucial as it keeps you from being taken down easily, and breaking your opponent's balance dramatically helps you to take him down. Leverage is important when the final action of the takedown is executed. For instance, for the sumo kimarite hip throw (koshinage) to be effective, your hips must be thrust against the front of your oppo-nent's hips so they become a fulcrum for the throw. This enables you to throw someone two times your size. Also mentioned earlier in chapter 2 is Mainoumi's preference for leg-tripping techniques, as they are a very effective way of toppling a much larger opponent. This is similar to the idea of chopping down a huge tree at its base to make it fall. Lever his leg out from under your opponent and let gravity do the rest. As seen earlier, the younger offshoots of sumo, jujitsu and judo, utilize these three concepts of movement, balance, and leverage to help their practitioners successfully engage larger opponents as well.

The smaller, weaker martial artists were forced to devise technical ways to defeat larger, stronger opponents. That is the way martial arts systems such as jujitsu were created over the centuries. The smaller, weaker martial artist ultimately used his weakness as a strength. In his book *The Gracie Way*, Kid Peligro relates that in the early days of BJJ, Helio Gracie refined the techniques and tactics of jiu-jitsu even more "by experimenting with different leverages and adjustments" to suit his frail body.[39] He compensated for his physical condi-tion by using his intellect. Without the innovative genius of Helio Gracie, the formidable martial art of Brazilian jiu-jitsu as we know it today would not exist.

From a sumo perspective, the popular and successful smaller rikishi Mainoumi used his weakness, his small stature, to his advantage. This forced him to employ up to thirty-three types of kimarite in his wrestling days, earning him his distinctive nickname, "Department Store of Techniques," as pointed out above. Recall also that a smaller rikishi usually has a belt-grabbing style of wrestling, which is a learned technical skill. Many times this belt-grabbing or clinching style neutralizes the usual power and speed-based pushing style used by larger rikishi. Just as in MMA, the clinch stops much of your opponent's striking ability.

Gladwell's book showed that by fighting unconventionally, not according to an opponent's rules, a small fighter greatly increases his chances of beating a giant. To paraphrase master grappler Gene LeBell: to do something illegal in a fighter's game, something he doesn't know, is the best way to beat any fighter. Underdog tactics are challenging.

In the beginning of modern MMA, small submission grapplers regularly beat larger opponents. Small submission grapplers, especially BJJ practitioners, fought unconventionally compared to the large strikers and Western wrestlers. The small submission grappler usually took the large striker down into the ground phase, pulling the striker out of his element and exactly where the submission grappler thrives. When facing the Western wrestler, the submission grappler would usually let the wrestler take him down and employ the guard from the bottom position, a position completely unfamiliar to Western wrestlers early on. A classic example of this is when Royce Gracie, a small BJJ fighter, submitted a much larger and stronger Western wrestler, Dan Severn, from the bottom guard position with a triangle choke in an early UFC fight. The small submission grapplers' special techniques and tactics hide their weaknesses, namely their lack of size and strength. To be a proficient submission grappler is a hard-won skill.

Now MMA fighters have evolved to become even more complete fighters. A "sprawl and brawl" fighter can thwart takedowns better than a one-dimensional striker, making the "ground and pound" and submission fighter's job of getting the fight to ground much more difficult. With Lyoto Machida's use of sumo in MMA as a "sprawl and brawl" fighter, he has neutralized many a fighter's ground game. Western wrestlers in MMA have learned to strike when on their feet and on the ground. This makes the submission fighter's job more difficult as avoiding heavy strikes from the bottom in the guard from a large wrestler is not easy. Now submission grapplers have adapted as well by including more striking and takedowns into their training.

Many top MMA fighters today are such well-rounded, complete fighters that there is a blurry line as to which of the three basic fighter categories they fall into. With this more complex field of fighters, the clinch phase is even more critical. As mentioned earlier in this chapter, the clinch phase is the hinge that connects the two other phases. Proficiency in the clinch gives you the huge advantage of dictating where the fight will lead: to the ground or staying on your feet. The clinch phase for many is a neglected skill set. Martial arts systems such as sumo, which enhance your clinch-phase skills, are even more important to know to be both competitive in MMA and effective in self-defense.

What Gladwell convincingly argues is that the attributes we perceive as strengths—great size and strength, for example—may well be ultimately weaknesses, while attributes we perceive as weaknesses, like small size and lack of strength, may well turn out to be strengths. What happens when we misinterpret our advantages or disadvantages? We do not make the right decisions. In MMA that could mean getting knocked out or submitted. The truth is found in training and competition. The more experience you have, the better your decisions will be.

Fighting spirit is not necessarily a matter of physical size but rather of psychological attitude. Often, it is not the biggest, strongest, or fastest fighter who is victorious in the end but the one who doesn't give up.

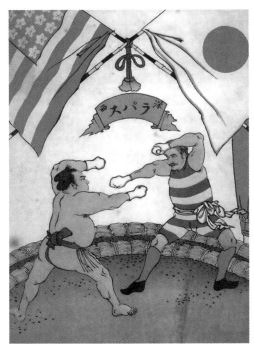

Woodblock print depicting a Japanese rikishi vs. an American sailor. The Japanese writing above the fighters on this old print translates to Western sparring or Western boxing. Meiji period, late nineteenth century.

(Author unknown, Wikimedia Commons.)

Physical Conditioning

Many consider physical conditioning to be the most important aspect of a martial artist's training regime. Techniques cannot be ideally applied without the support of a well-conditioned body. Professional rikishi and mixed martial artists also have something else in common: their physical conditioning is on par with the top athletes in the world. Of course, their conditioning programs differ as the goals of each of these combat sports are very different. Strength, endurance, and flexibility, the major elements of physical conditioning, are addressed vigorously in both sumo and MMA. Because a sumo match rarely lasts more than a minute, endurance training is not as critical as in an MMA contest where there are typically up to three to five rounds that are five minutes each. Strength and explosiveness are more important in a sumo match, and sumo physical conditioning is done with this in mind.

Because the most apparent physical link between sumo and MMA is the clinch phase, what are the physical requirements for this special phase of combat? According to experts Renzo Gracie and John Danaher, the physical requirements for locking up into the clinch phase of combat are "balance, gripping strength, and driving power."[40] Core stability and sensitivity are needed for balance, gripping and pulling conditioning are needed for gripping strength, and leg conditioning is needed for driving power. By strongly improving in these three areas, you are on your way to having a better clinch game.

Conquering Fear: Development of Courage in Soldiers and Other High Risk Occupations by Halim Ozkaptan, PhD, with General Crosbie E. Saint, Ret., and Colonel Robert S. Fiero, Ret., thoroughly examines the connection between physical fitness and the psychological will to conquer fear and perform the task at hand under adverse conditions.[41] Success in battle tomorrow grows from today's hard work. Being out of endurance can make even the strongest afraid. The warrior's fortitude begins with his physical conditioning, fortitude being the emotional strength to press on against great obstacles. The mind-body connection is crucial to understand if one is to conquer fear and perform effectively under extreme pressure.

This outstanding quote by Alexander the Great's chief physician reiterates the importance of this mind-body connection. "Without Knowledge, Skill cannot be focused. Without Skill, Strength cannot be brought to bear and without Strength, Knowledge may not be applied."[42] This quote not only expresses the circular flow of these attributes but also implies that they amplify each other in an ever-increasing beneficial spiral. Although the main focus of this book is on the physical techniques of sumo, it is critical to grasp and apply the elements that support and enhance these techniques. This is especially important when smaller warriors take on larger opponents.

Sumo and MMA Conclusion

In this chapter we viewed sumo from an MMA perspective. We saw that the over-under clinch is the most common form of clinch in both sumo and MMA. We also explored the reasons an MMA fighter would want to go to the ground phase with takedowns. No matter what type of MMA fighter you are—"sprawl and brawl" fighter, submission grappler, or "ground and pound" fighter—sumo skills as shown here can give you a definite edge. We revealed in some detail how the well-rounded and successful MMA fighter Lyoto "The Dragon" Machida made sumo part of his MMA toolbox in a brilliant way. Finally, we briefly discussed physical conditioning as a crucial element in your training regime. The next chapter will show in many useful pictures selected sumo techniques from an MMA perspective you could easily add to your martial arts arsenal.

CHAPTER 4

Technical Photos

Introduction

In this final chapter, we illustrate many selected sumo techniques from an MMA perspective that can be easily integrated into your martial arts game. First, for your safety while training, breakfalls will be shown. Second, the proper fighting stance will be examined for MMA compared to sumo. Third, supplementary techniques will be demonstrated to help you with sumo's winning moves, kimarite. Finally, we will examine in depth selected kimarite that are highly applicable to fighting and MMA. This final chapter ties together everything presented in this book so you will have an excellent understanding of how sumo can be used in MMA and other grappling situations.

Here are some important tips to follow when performing the takedowns in this chapter. It is best to attack with combinations. Just as a boxer strings punches together looking for the knockout, so the takedown specialist combines takedown attempts to enter the ground phase. The first takedown should be a committed attack so you get the right reaction for the second takedown attack. One committed technique flows from the next until victory is achieved. Also, proper transition from clinch-phase takedowns to the ground phase involves staying close to your opponent as you follow up immediately with ground techniques. If there is too much distance between you and your opponent after your successful takedown, you will almost certainly lose the advantage of your takedown.

Breakfalls (Ukemi)

Ukemi literally means "receiving body." It is the art of knowing how to respond properly to an attack so the receiver is not injured. Often these skills resemble tumbling and are practiced in many Japanese martial arts, not just in sumo. The primary objective in breakfalls is to protect your head and spine, which house your delicate nervous system. When done properly, breakfalls soften blows to the bones and joints. Breakfalls significantly lessen the amount of damage sustained in a fall. The force of the fall is distributed over noncritical areas of the body. Knowing how to breakfall is not only important when being thrown by your opponent but also in daily life. Many accidents involve falling down, whether it is from a trip or slip. In the martial arts, being able to inflict punishment is important, but being able to receive it can be even more critical.

For training safety, practice your takedowns and breakfalls on a good padded surface to help prevent unwanted injuries. When first practicing breakfalls, start slow and start low. It is always advisable to begin from a lying-down position to get the correct body position. Then progressively move to a sitting position, to a crouching position, and finally to a standing position. In the beginning all rolls should be started from a kneeling position. When performing rear and sideways breakfalls, you will be slapping out with both arms or just one arm. Therefore, your arms should be spread at a forty-five-degree angle from your body. This spread keeps you from landing directly on your arm with your body. It also keeps the shoulder joint from absorbing too much pressure if the spread is too wide. Finally, make sure you tuck your chin into your chest when instructed, so you protect the back of your head from hitting the floor.

Forward Breakfall (Mae Ukemi)

Forward Breakfall (Mae Ukemi) kneeling

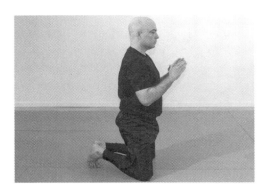

Andrew starts on his knees.

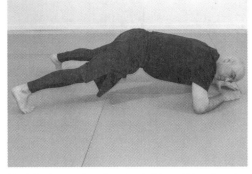

He falls forward and protects himself by slapping out and supporting himself with his arms. He makes contact on the ground from his fingertips to his elbows all at once to spread the impact of the fall across a wide surface area. Before he makes contact with his arms on the ground, he twists his face to the side just in case his arms cannot stop the full impact and his head hits the ground. Twisting his face to the side protects his nose, mouth, and eyes if his head makes contact with the ground. After the fall, Andrew makes contact with the ground only with his toes and forearms to protect the trunk of his body.

Forward Breakfall (Mae Ukemi) standing

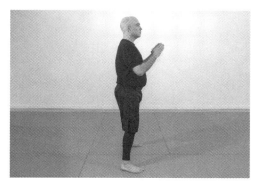

Andrew starts with a standing position.

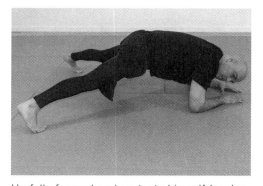

He falls forward and protects himself by slapping out and supporting himself with his arms. He makes contact on the ground from his fingertips to his elbows all at once to spread the impact of the fall across a wide surface area. Before he makes contact with his arms on the ground, he twists his face to the side just in case his arms cannot stop the full impact and his head hits the ground. Twisting his face to the side protects his nose, mouth, and eyes if his head makes contact with the ground. After the fall, Andrew makes contact with the ground only with his toes and forearms to protect the trunk of his body.

Rear Breakfall (Ushiro Ukemi)

Rear Breakfall (Ushiro Ukemi) squatting

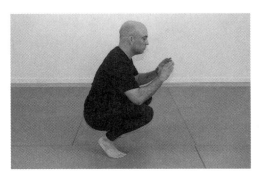

Andrew starts with a squatting position.

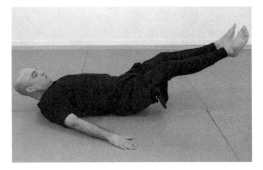

He falls backward while tucking his chin to his chest to protect his head from the backward impact on the ground. Just before his back hits the ground, Andrew slaps out with both arms making contact on the ground from fingertips to elbows all at the same time to spread the impact of the fall across a wide surface area. Andrew's arms should be spread at a forty-five-degree angle from his body. This spread keeps him from landing directly on his arms with his body. It also keeps his shoulder joint from absorbing too much pressure if the spread is too wide.

Rear Breakfall (Ushiro Ukemi) standing

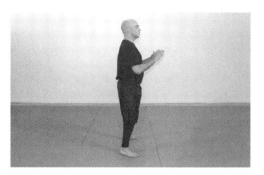

Andrew starts with a standing position.

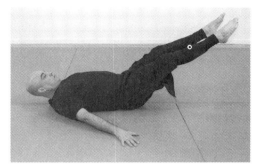

He falls backward while tucking his chin to his chest to protect his head from the backward impact on the ground. Just before his back hits the ground, Andrew slaps out with both arms making contact on the ground from finger-tips to elbows all at the same time to spread the impact of the fall across a wide surface area. Andrew's arms should be spread at a forty-five-degree angle from his body. This spread keeps him from landing directly on his arms with his body. It also keeps his shoulder joint from absorbing too much pressure if the spread is too wide.

Side Breakfall (Yoko Ukemi)

Side Breakfall (Yoko Ukemi) lying down

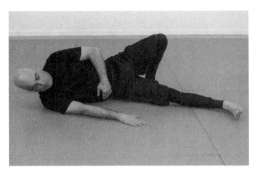

Andrew starts by lying down on the ground.

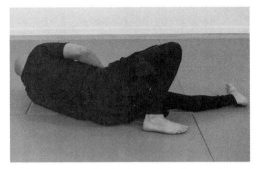

Andrew rotates his body to the other side and slaps out with his lower arm. He falls to the side while tucking his chin to his chest to protect his head from the sideways impact on the ground. Andrew slaps out with one arm making contact on the ground from fingertips to elbow all at the same time to spread the impact of the fall across a wide surface area. Andrew's arm should be spread at a forty-five-degree angle from his body. This spread keeps him from landing directly on his arm with his body. It also keeps his shoulder joint from absorbing too much pressure if the spread is too wide. Andrew can once again rotate to the other side, repeating the breakfall.

Side Breakfall (Yoko Ukemi) standing

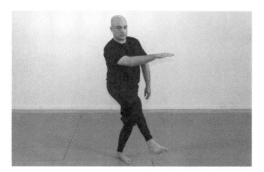

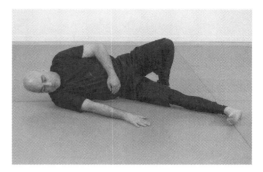

Andrew starts with a standing position. Andrew swings his right leg to his left to begin the breakfall. He readies his right arm as well by extending it and swinging it to his left.

Andrew lowers his body with his left leg and falls to his right. He slaps the ground with his right arm just before his body hits the ground. He falls to the side while tucking his chin to his chest to protect his head from the sideways impact on the ground. Andrew slaps out with one arm making contact on the ground from fingertips to elbow all at the same time to spread the impact of the fall across a wide surface area. Andrew's arm should be spread at a forty-five-degree angle from his body. This spread keeps him from landing directly on his arm with his body. It also keeps his shoulder joint from absorbing too much pressure if the spread is too wide.

Forward-Rolling Breakfall (Mae Mawari Ukemi)

Forward-Rolling Breakfall (Mae Mawari Ukemi) kneeling

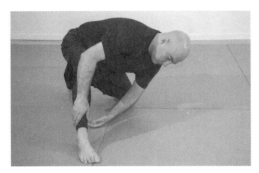 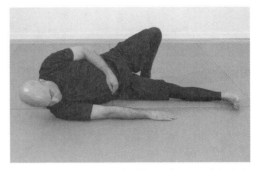

Andrew starts with kneeling on his left knee. He brings his left arm between his legs and tucks in his chin to his chest to protect his head.

Andrew rolls from his fingertips to his left shoulder to his right hip in a smooth diagonal path across his back. He slaps the ground with his right arm to dissipate the fall. Andrew slaps out with his right arm making contact on the ground with his arm from fingertips to elbow all at the same time to spread the impact of the fall across a wide surface area. Andrew's right arm should be spread at a forty-five-degree angle from his body. This spread keeps him from landing directly on his arm with his body. It also keeps his shoulder joint from absorbing too much pressure if the spread is too wide. He ends up on the ground on his right side.

Forward-Rolling Breakfall (Mae Mawari Ukemi) standing

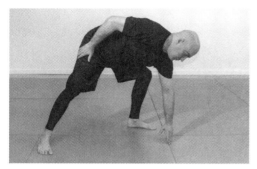 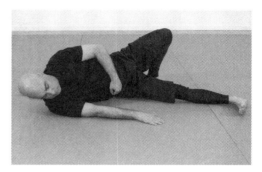

Andrew starts with a standing position. He brings his left arm between his legs and tucks in his chin to his chest to protect his head.

Andrew rolls from his fingertips to his left shoulder to his right hip in a smooth, diagonal path across his back. He slaps the ground with his right arm to dissipate the fall. Andrew slaps out with his right arm making contact on the ground from fingertips to elbow all at the same time to spread the impact of the fall across a wide surface area. Andrew's arm should be spread at a forty-five-degree angle from his body. This spread keeps him from landing directly on his arm with his body. It also keeps his shoulder joint from absorbing too much pressure if the spread is too wide. He ends up on the ground on his right side.

Sumo and MMA Fighting Stances

The squatting low stance with the hands held low in sumo is not suitable for MMA fighters as mobility and protection from headhunting strikes are required for success in MMA. Therefore, the stance that will be used in the free-movement phase will be the typical boxer's stance. As stated by experts Renzo Gracie and John Danaher, the boxer's stance gives you the mobility and head protection needed in MMA. "Small variations in stance are certainly acceptable. However, the core ideas behind an efficient fighting stance—the hands up to protect the head, feet slightly more than shoulder-width apart, the weight evenly distributed on the balls of the feet, the rear heel slightly off the floor, the chin tucked down, the elbows in, the knees bent—these are common to all."[43]

Sumo Fighting Stance

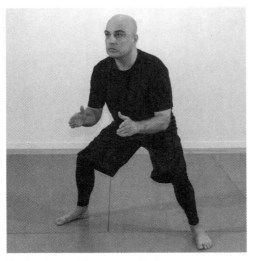 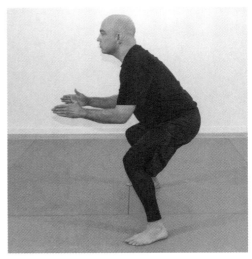

Notice the wide stance that gives you good balance but bad mobility.

Also the hands are low, which is not good for protecting your head from strikes.

MMA Fighting Stance

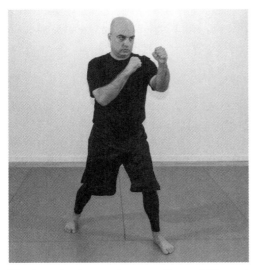 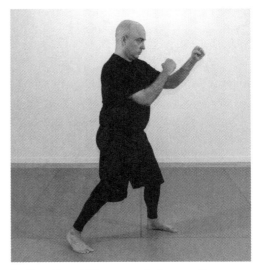

The boxer's stance gives you the mobility and head protection needed in MMA.

Notice the differences between the sumo fighting stance and the MMA fighting stance.

Supplementary Techniques

While these supplementary techniques may not be complete winning moves in sumo (kimarite), they can help make the kimarite much more effective. Being able to execute an underhook properly is a crucial skill in setting up many of these kimarite. As mentioned in the earlier chapters, fighting for inside control is a constant battle in the clinch phase. These supplementary techniques will help you in this battle.

Grips

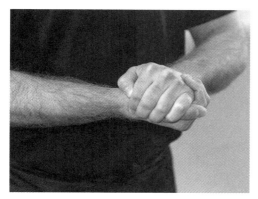

Palm-to-palm grip.

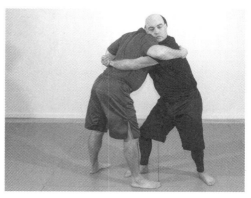

The palm-to-palm grip is very useful when your opponent is not much larger than you.

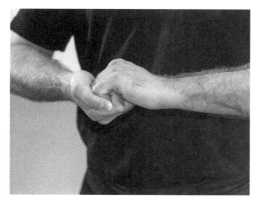

S-grip.

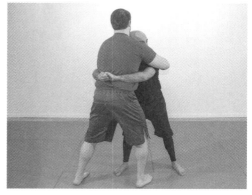

The S-grip is often needed when your opponent is much larger than you.

Over-Under Clinch

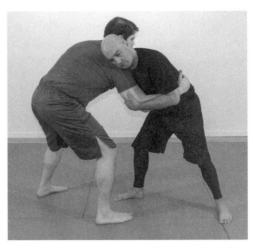

The author, Andrew (right), secures the over-under clinch on his training partner, Dave. For this book, it is critical to understand the over-under clinch, as most of the technical photos start from this position. The over-under clinch is the most commonly used clinch in both sumo and MMA.

Underhook Technique

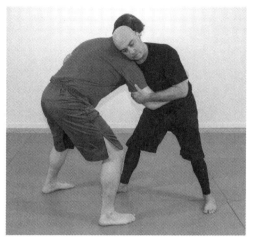

Andrew (right) and Dave lock up in the over-under clinch.

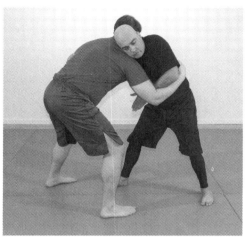

Andrew swims his left overhook into the natural gap in the crook of Dave's right elbow.

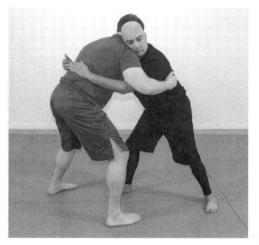

Andrew finishes this movement into a left underhook for inside control.

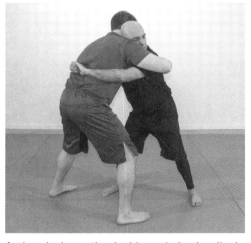

Andrew locks on the double-underhooks clinch. This technique is important to grasp as it is a movement that is used often in this book's technical photos.

Over-Under Clinch Exercise

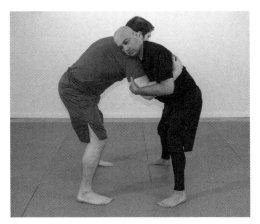 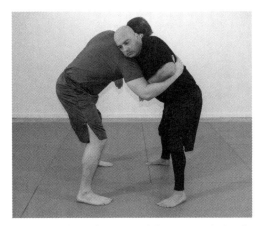

Andrew and Dave begin in the over-under clinch, but this time to simplify the exercise, their stances are parallel to each other. While doing this exercise, your legs don't change positions.

Andrew swims his overhook into an underhook, and at the same time, Dave does the same thing on his side. Also, Andrew and Dave switch where they place their heads, so in the end, their heads rest on the side where their training partner has his underhook.

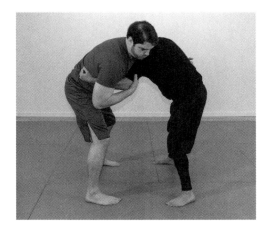

So after one cycle of underhooks, they are in an opposite-sided over-under clinch. Multiple cycles of this exercise with varying degrees of resistance can be performed. One game you can play is for each person to try to get double-underhooks. It is a great way to warm up before a grappling workout.

Push Escape from the Over-Under Clinch

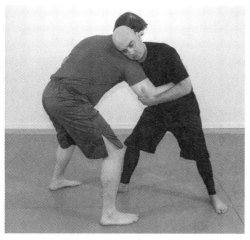

Andrew (right) and Dave begin in the over-under clinch (right legs forward).

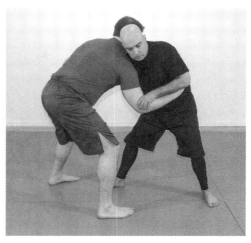

Andrew presses Dave's right underhook down at the crook of the elbow with his left overhook hand. This disengages Dave's underhook.

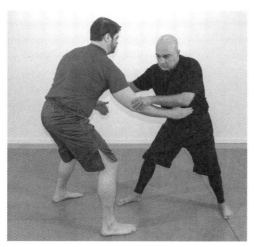

Andrew then disengages his underhook so he can press on Dave's chest to fully get out of the over-under clinch.

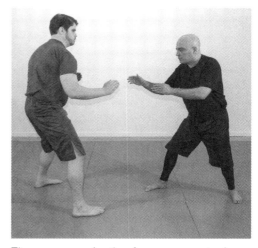

They are now in the free-movement phase. This is a BJJ technique, but it has definite relevance in sumo and MMA.

Push Escape from the Double-Underhooks Clinch, Two Ways

Palms Push Escape

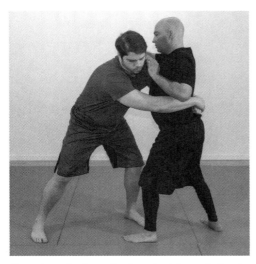 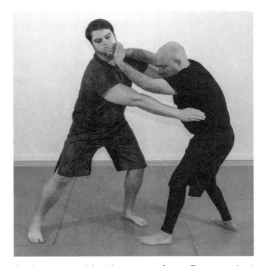

Dave has Andrew in the double-underhooks clinch.

Andrew sags his hips away from Dave and at the same time pushes strongly on Dave's chin with both of his palms to escape the double-underhooks clinch. This chin push escape only works well if you start it before your attacker fully locks on the double-underhooks clinch; if you start it too late, you won't have the leverage to do it. This is a BJJ technique, but it has definite relevance in sumo and MMA.

Frame Push Escape

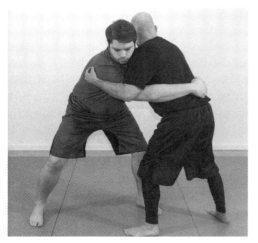

Dave has Andrew in the double-underhooks clinch.

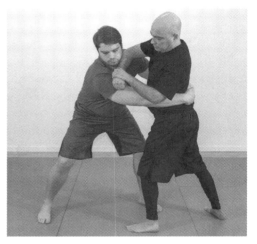

Andrew begins to make a frame with his arms by sinking his right forearm under Dave's chin on his throat. Andrew grabs his right arm at the wrist with his left hand to support it.

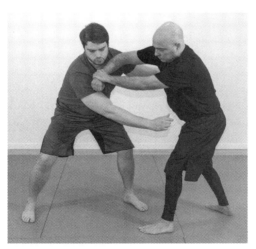

Andrew presses into Dave's throat with his framed arms. The area closer to his elbow is used to press into Dave in order to employ the full force of his body against Dave. Andrew continues the pressing motion while he sags his hips away from Dave to escape the double-underhooks clinch. This is a BJJ technique, but it has definite relevance in sumo and MMA.

Kimarite: Sumo's Winning Moves

There are currently eighty-two kimarite (sumo's winning moves) recognized by the Japan Sumo Association. For this chapter of technical photos, forty-eight kimarite will be demonstrated. These forty-eight kimarite were specially selected for their usefulness in MMA competition. The kimarite that rely heavily on a belt grip to work are not included in this chapter as they are not practical for the MMA fighter. Most of the kimarite in the photos can be easily modified for MMA to throw down your opponent without a belt grip by using controlling body locks like an overhook or underhook.

It is definitely not necessary to be very proficient in all of these forty-eight kimarite. Even in the extreme case of the popular and successful rikishi Mainoumi, "Department Store of Techniques," he used up to thirty-three types of kimarite in his wrestling career. As shown in the sumo case studies section of this book, most rikishi have several favorite techniques (*tokui waza*) that they use frequently because they find them particularly effective. Even in MMA, most successful fighters have favorite or preferred techniques in all the phases of fighting: free-movement phase, clinch phase, and ground phase. It is always better to focus hard on training a small number of techniques that suit your body type and fighting goals than to dabble in many techniques and be much less proficient in them especially when facing tough, determined opponents.

When it comes to the defenses against these kimarite, knowing they exist is the first line of defense. You will fall easy prey to these kimarite if you do not have any knowledge of them. Knowing what to expect gives you a great advantage. Interrupting the application of the kimarite is the best strategy. Maintaining inside control and your balance are the basics of thwarting many kimarite. These hard-won skills come with proper practice.

Basic Techniques (Kihonwaza)

Kimarite basic techniques of pushing and thrusting are the fundamental tried-and-true moves that work the most often in sumo. However, these moves ideally require speed and power, and that makes them less effective for a smaller player. As discussed earlier, a smaller rikishi usually has a belt-grabbing style of wrestling, which is a learned technical skill. This belt-grabbing or clinching style many times neutralizes the usual power and speed-based pushing and thrusting style used by larger rikishi. As in MMA, the clinch stops much of your opponent's striking ability.

Front Push Out (Oshidashi)

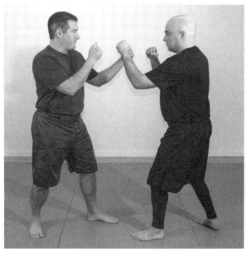

Andrew and Matt face each other in MMA fighting stances (left legs forward).

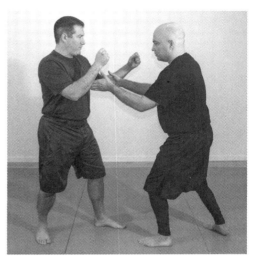

Andrew pushes Matt.

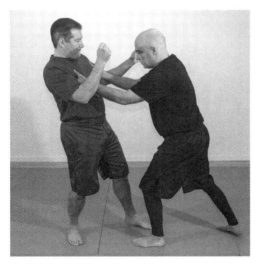

Unlike a front thrust out (tsukidashi), Andrew must maintain hand contact at all times. Pushing (oshi) is the most fundamental tried-and-true sumo technique.

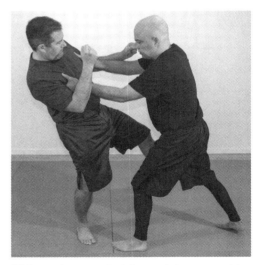

Slide or step your feet forward, keep your hips low, and be sure to make contact when pushing with the pinky-side edge of your palm to conduct the most energy into your opponent. This technique is useful when you want to move your opponent for varied reasons.

Front Push Down (Oshitaoshi)

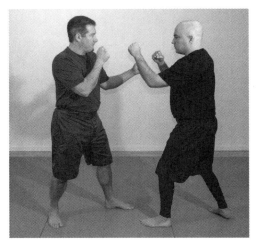

Andrew and Matt face each other in MMA fighting stances (left legs forward).

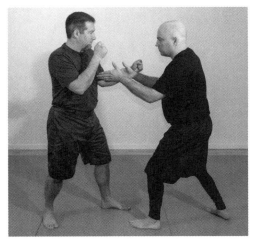

Andrew begins to push Matt to the ground.

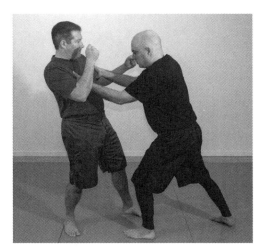

Unlike a front thrust down (tsukitaoshi), Andrew must maintain hand contact at all times. Pushing (oshi) is the most fundamental tried-and-true sumo technique.

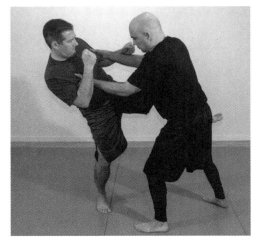

Slide or step your feet forward, keep your hips low, and be sure to make contact when pushing with the pinky-side edge of your palm to conduct the most energy into your opponent.

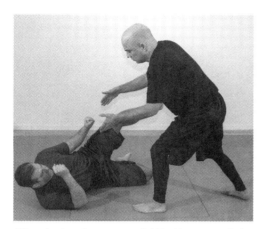

After Andrew's opponent hits the ground, he is sure to follow up immediately with ground techniques.

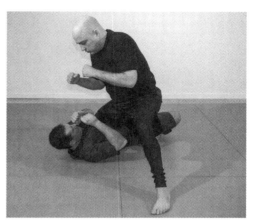

If there is too much separation between Andrew and his opponent after grounding him, Andrew is probably going to lose the advantage.

Front Thrust Out (Tsukidashi)

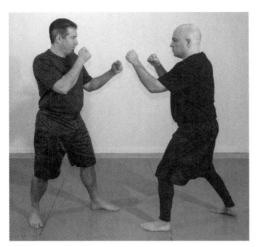 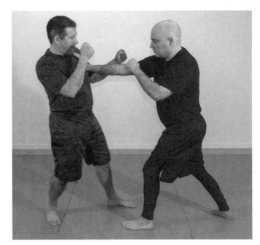

Andrew and Matt face each other in MMA fighting stances (left legs forward).

Andrew drives Matt backward with a constant rhythm of thrusting motions. Unlike the front push out, Andrew does not have to maintain hand contact at all times.

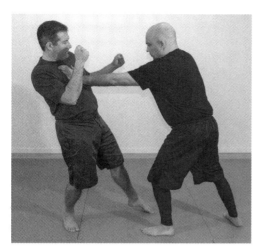 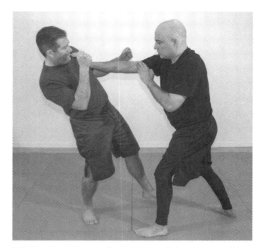

Like pushing, thrusting is one of the most fundamental tried-and-true techniques in sumo. To work optimally, this technique requires a constant fast windmill-like rotation of thrusts from both hands.

Slide or step your feet forward, keep your hips low, and be sure to make contact when thrusting with the pinky-side edge of your palm (not your fingers) to conduct the most energy into your opponent. The side you are sliding or stepping with is the same side as your arm thrust, so you put your weight behind them. The thrusting target is your opponent's chest, his center of mass, in an upward rising motion to uproot your opponent. This technique is useful when you want to move your opponent for varied reasons.

Front Thrust Down (Tsukitaoshi)

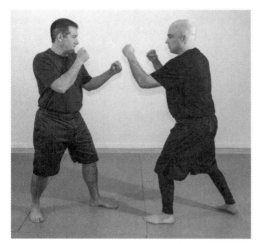 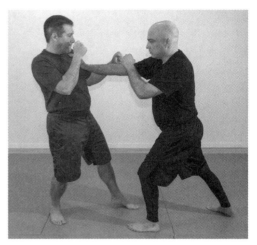

Andrew and Matt face each other in MMA fighting stances (left legs forward).

Andrew drives Matt backward with a constant rhythm of thrusting motions that causes Matt to fall to the ground. Unlike the front push down, Andrew does not have to maintain hand contact at all times.

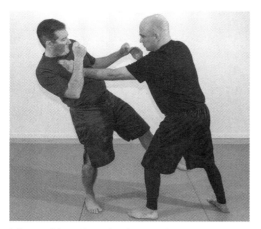 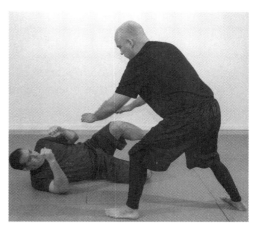

Like pushing, thrusting is one of the most funda-mental tried-and-true techniques in sumo. This technique works best with a constant fast windmill-like rotation of thrusts from both hands. Slide or step your feet forward, keep your hips low, and be sure to make contact when thrusting with the pinky-side edge of your palm (not your fingers) to conduct the most energy into your opponent. The side you are sliding or stepping with is the same side as your arm thrust, so you put your weight behind them. The thrusting target is your opponent's chest, his center of mass, in an upward rising motion to uproot your opponent.

After Andrew's opponent hits the ground, he is sure to follow up immediately with ground techniques.

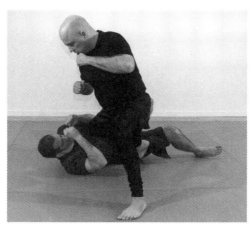

If there is too much separation between Andrew and his opponent after grounding him, Andrew is probably going to lose the advantage.

Throwing Techniques (Nagete)

To work best, kimarite throwing techniques require that your opponent pushes into you. Throws differ from takedowns in the manner in which your opponent is grounded. Throws tend to slam your opponent down with a high-altitude trajectory while takedowns are not as flashy in that they focus on simply grounding your opponent and getting a dominant ground position.

One-Arm Shoulder Throw (Ipponzeoi)

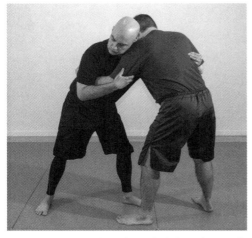 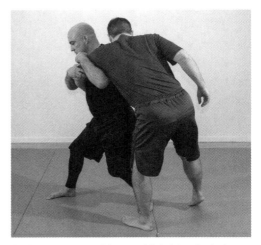

From the over-under clinch (left legs forward), Matt pushes.

Andrew opens up his rear (right) leg for balance as he turns his hips away from Matt by pivoting on both of his feet. At the same time, Andrew disengages his left underhook.

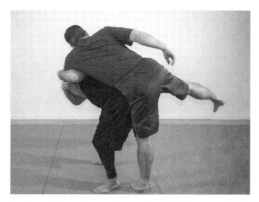

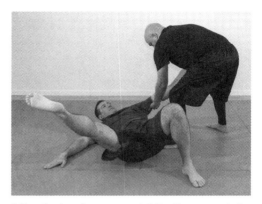

Andrew then steps forward with his rear (left) leg, previously his front leg. Andrew goes with this push and pulls Matt's left underhook with both of his arms as he turns his back to him with his hips sunk in under his opponent in order to throw him over his shoulder or hip.

After Andrew's opponent hits the ground, he is sure to follow up immediately with ground techniques.

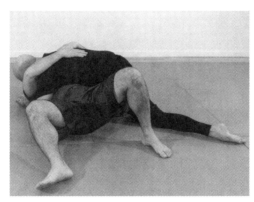

If there is too much separation between Andrew and his opponent after grounding him, Andrew is probably going to lose the advantage.

Hooking Inner-Thigh Throw (Kakenage)

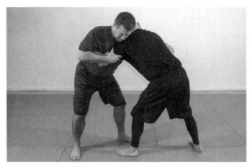

From the over-under clinch (left legs forward) Matt pushes.

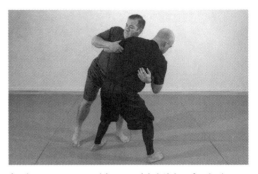

Andrew opens up his rear (right) leg for balance as he turns his hips away from Matt by pivoting on both feet.

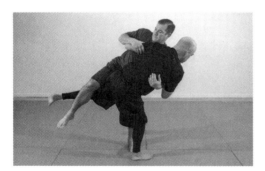

Andrew's left leg now hooks Matt's right leg at the inner thigh. Andrew lifts his left leg to break Matt's balance. Andrew brings Matt to a lower level while quickly and strongly lifting his left leg. If your first throwing attempt does not work, you can hop on your supporting right leg while continuously trying to throw.

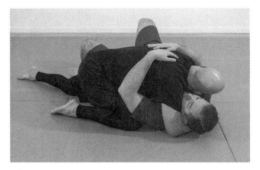

After Andrew's opponent hits the ground, he is sure to follow up immediately with ground techniques. If there is too much separation between Andrew and his opponent after grounding him, Andrew is probably going to lose the advantage.

Hip Throw (Koshinage)

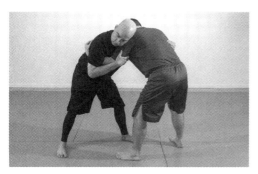

From the over-under clinch (left legs forward), Matt pushes.

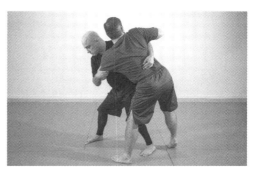

Andrew opens up his rear (right) leg for balance when he turns his hips away from Matt by pivoting on both feet.

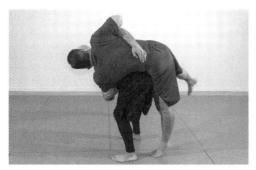

Andrew then steps forward with his rear (left) leg, previously his front leg. Andrew goes with this push and turns his back to him with his hips sunk in under his opponent in order to throw him over his hip.

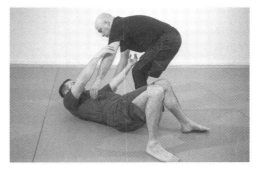

Andrew throws Matt over his hip. After Andrew's opponent hits the ground, he is sure to follow up immediately with ground techniques.

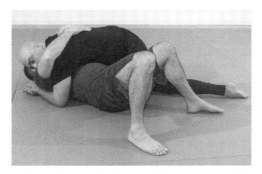

If there is too much separation between Andrew and his opponent after grounding him, Andrew is probably going to lose the advantage.

Armlock Throw (Kotenage)

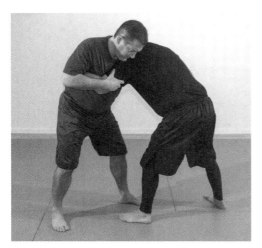 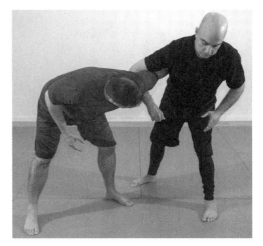

From the over-under clinch (left legs forward), Matt pushes.

Andrew goes with this push and sinks his right overhook deeply onto Matt's left elbow. At the same time, he fully steps back with his front (left) leg and twists his hips to the left in order to lower Matt's head and torso.

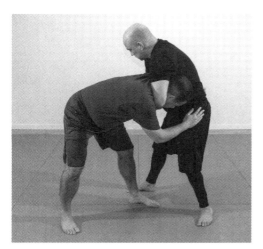

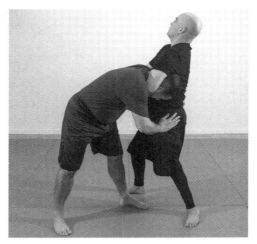

With his disengaged left arm, Andrew sinks in a BJJ–style head and arm guillotine choke to finish off his opponent.

This kimarite is so powerful that many rikishi injure their opponent's arms. This kimarite was modified to end in an MMA submission rather than a throw.

Headlock Throw (Kubinage)

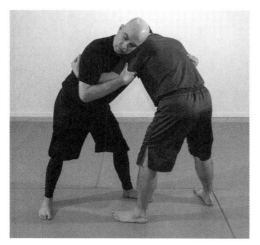 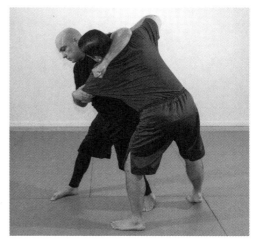

From the over-under clinch (left legs forward), Matt pushes.

Andrew opens up his rear (right) leg for balance when he turns his hips away from Matt by pivoting on both feet. At the same time, Andrew goes with this push and disengages his left underhook to swing it tightly around Matt's neck.

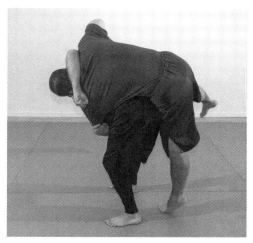

Andrew then steps forward with his rear (left) leg, previously his front leg. Andrew turns into Matt to get his hips under him. He throws Matt by extending his legs, pulling down Matt's head and tightly pulling down his overhook on the far arm.

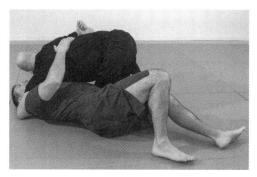

After Andrew's opponent hits the ground, he is sure to follow up immediately with ground techniques.

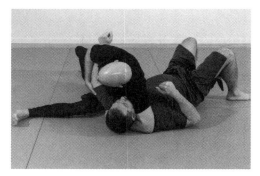

If there is too much separation between Andrew and his opponent after grounding him, Andrew is probably going to lose the advantage.

Body-Drop Throw (Nichonage)

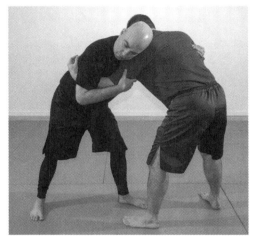

From the over-under clinch (left legs forward), Matt pushes.

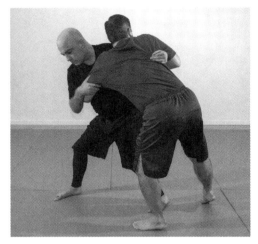

Andrew opens up his rear (right) leg for balance when he turns his hips away from Matt by pivoting on both feet.

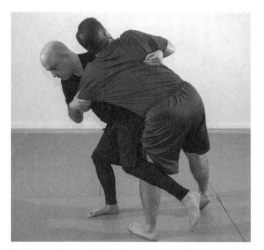

Andrew places his left leg at the knee against the outside of Matt's left leg and sweeps it.

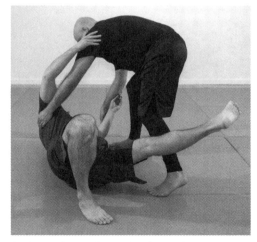

Andrew also pulls and twists with his upper body so Matt is thrown over his left leg. After Andrew's opponent hits the ground, he is sure to follow up immediately with ground techniques.

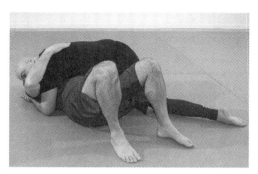

If there is too much separation between Andrew and his opponent after grounding him, Andrew is probably going to lose the advantage.

Beltless Arm Throw (Sukuinage)

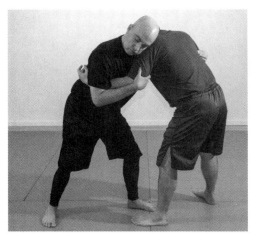 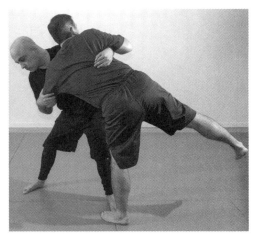

From the over-under clinch (left legs forward), Matt pushes.

Andrew opens up his rear (right) leg for balance when he turns his hips away from Matt by pivoting on both feet.

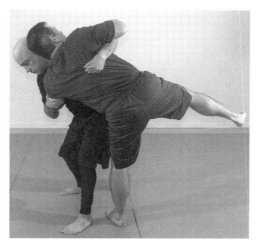

Andrew then steps forward with his rear (left) leg, previously his front leg. Andrew twists his upper body hold away from Matt and continues to step strongly forward with his hips and left leg to throw Matt.

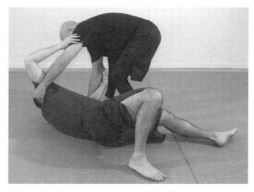

After Andrew's opponent hits the ground, he is sure to follow up immediately with ground techniques.

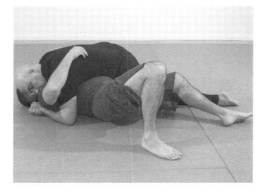

If there is too much separation between Andrew and his opponent after grounding him, Andrew is probably going to lose the advantage.

Inner-Thigh-Lift Throw (Yaguranage)

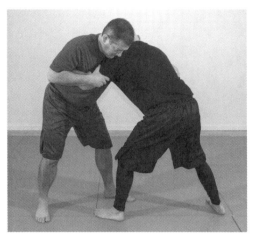

From the over-under clinch (left legs forward), Matt pushes.

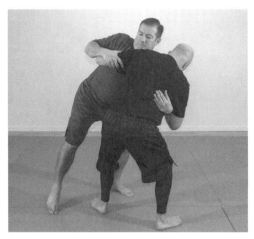

Andrew opens up his rear (right) leg for balance when he turns his hips away from Matt by pivoting on both feet.

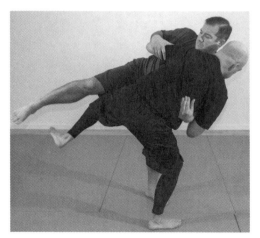

Andrew's left leg at the outside of his knee lifts Matt's right inner thigh. Andrew and Matt are chest to chest. Andrew lifts his left leg to break Matt's balance. Andrew brings Matt to a lower level while quickly and strongly lifting his left leg. Andrew lifts with his knee and pulls with his upper body for the throw.

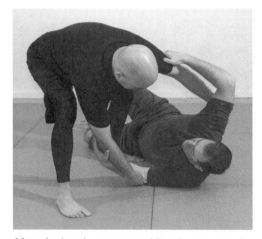

After Andrew's opponent hits the ground, he is sure to follow up immediately with ground techniques.

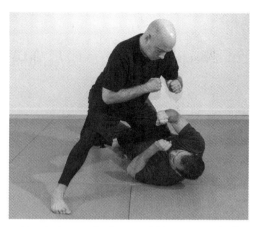

If there is too much separation between Andrew and his opponent after grounding him, Andrew is probably going to lose the advantage.

Leg-Tripping Techniques (Kakete)

Kimarite leg-tripping techniques mostly require that your opponent's lead leg is well forward and your opponent is fading back so the lead leg has less weight on it and you can capitalize on that. In chapter 2 we saw that a successful smaller sumo player preferred leg-tripping techniques as they are an excellent way of taking down larger opponents. Therefore, in this section a larger opponent will be used to help illustrate this.

Leg Pick (Ashitori)

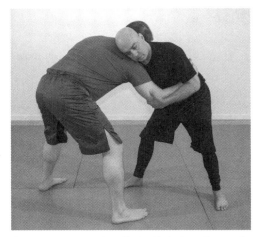 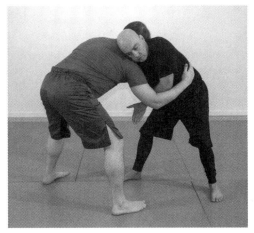

From the over-under clinch (right legs forward), Dave pulls Andrew, which makes Dave's front leg lighter.

Andrew swims his left overhook into a left underhook to get inside control.

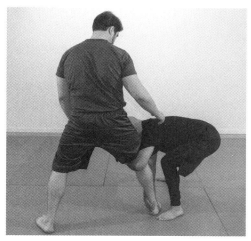

At the same time, Andrew fully steps forward with his rear leg to the outside in order to grab and elevate Dave's front leg at the knee and ankle.

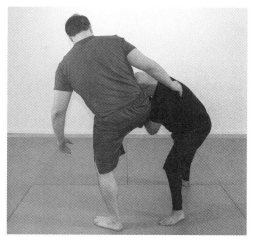

When Andrew goes to take Dave's leg, he squats low so that he uses his hips to elevate the leg, not just his arms.

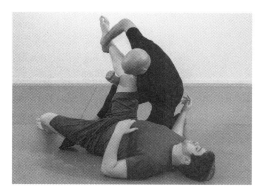

He steps back with his lead (left) leg to take him down. After Andrew's opponent hits the ground, he is sure to follow up immediately with ground techniques.

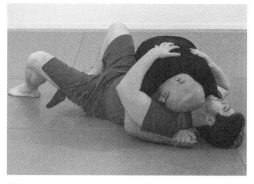

If there is too much separation between Andrew and his opponent after grounding him, Andrew is probably going to lose the advantage.

Pulling Heel Hook (Chongake)

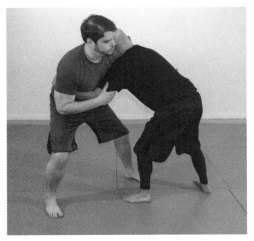

From the over-under clinch (left legs forward), Dave pulls Andrew, which makes Dave's front leg lighter.

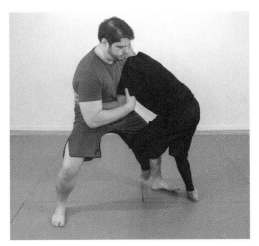

With his lead (left) leg, Andrew hooks Dave's lead (left) leg heel to heel from the inside. Andrew leans into Dave while pulling his heel hook, which sends Dave to the ground.

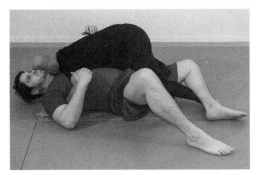

After Andrew's opponent hits the ground, he is sure to follow up immediately with ground techniques.

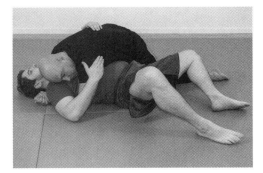

If there is too much separation between Andrew and his opponent after grounding him, Andrew is probably going to lose the advantage.

Inside Foot Sweep (Kekaeshi)

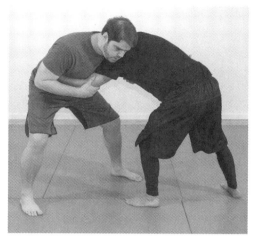

From the over-under clinch (left legs forward), Dave pulls Andrew, which makes Dave's front leg lighter.

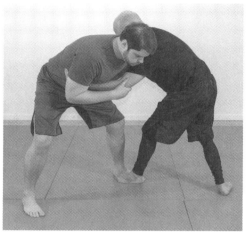

Andrew sweeps Dave's front (left) leg with his front (left) leg from the inside left to right.

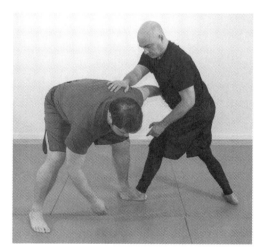

Andrew does a well-timed slap with his right hand on Dave's back to help the sweep take effect. After Andrew's opponent hits the ground, he is sure to follow up immediately with ground techniques.

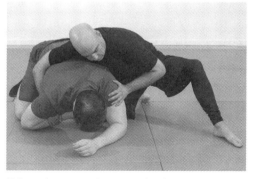

If there is too much separation between Andrew and his opponent after grounding him, Andrew is probably going to lose the advantage.

Twisting Backward Knee Trip (Kirikaeshi)

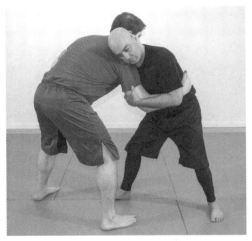

From the over-under clinch (right legs forward), Dave pulls.

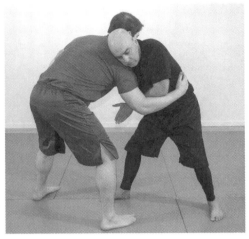

Andrew swims his left overhook into a left underhook to get the double-underhooks clinch while clasping his hands together.

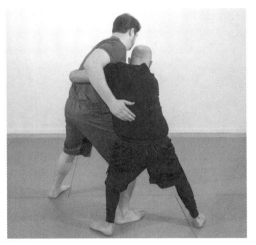

At the same time, he goes with the pull to fully enter in behind Dave with his rear leg so his left knee is positioned behind Dave's front leg.

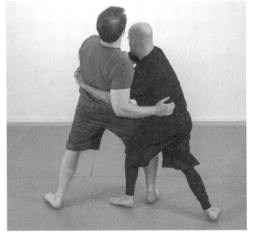

After twisting with his hips and upper body to his left, Andrew throws Dave over his front knee. After Andrew's opponent hits the ground, he is sure to follow up immediately with ground techniques.

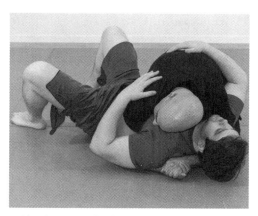

If there is too much separation between Andrew and his opponent after grounding him, Andrew is probably going to lose the advantage. This technique can be done without performing the double-underhooks clinch. Just clasp your hands together while in the over-under clinch, and perform the twisting backward knee trip. However, linking your hands together while in the over-under clinch may be difficult if your opponent is much larger than you.

Inside Thigh Scoop (Komatasukui)

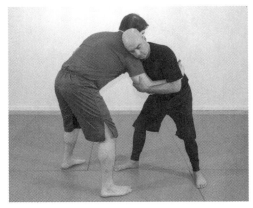

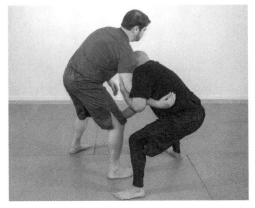

From the over-under clinch (right legs forward), Dave pulls Andrew, which makes Dave's front leg lighter.

Andrew capitalizes on this by fully stepping in with his rear leg and lifting Dave's front leg from the inside on or near the thigh with his disengaged right underhook arm.

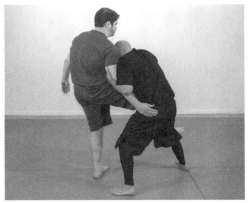

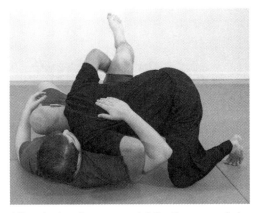

Andrew grips Dave's right arm tightly with his left overhook for control and buries his head and shoulder into Dave's shoulder and chest. When Andrew goes to take Dave's leg, he squats low so that he uses his hips to elevate the leg, not just his arms. Dave is then driven onto his back.

After Andrew's opponent hits the ground, he is sure to follow up immediately with ground techniques.

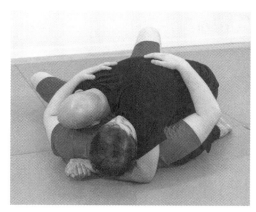

If there is too much separation between Andrew and his opponent after grounding him, Andrew is probably going to lose the advantage.

Triple-Attack Force Out (Mitokorozeme)

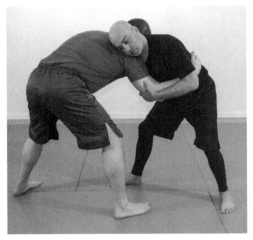

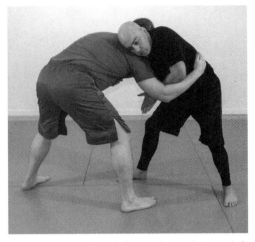

From the over-under clinch (right legs forward), Dave pulls.

Andrew swims his left overhook into a left underhook.

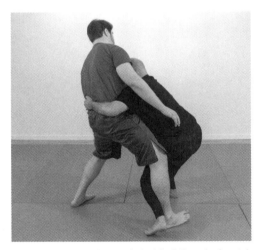

He enters in fully with his rear leg and places it behind Dave's front leg. By using three driving forces—the leg trip, right hand on Dave's left thigh, and his shoulder or head on Dave's chest or stomach—Andrew forces Dave onto his back. This is the potent kimarite that Mainoumi used to take down Akebono.

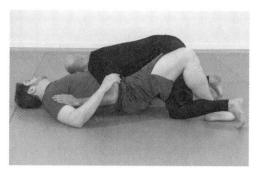

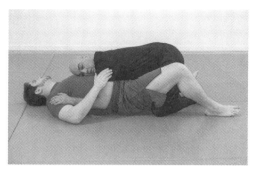

After Andrew's opponent hits the ground, he is sure to follow up immediately with ground techniques.

If there is too much separation between Andrew and his opponent after grounding him, Andrew is probably going to lose the advantage.

Ankle-Sweep Twist Down (Nimaigeri)

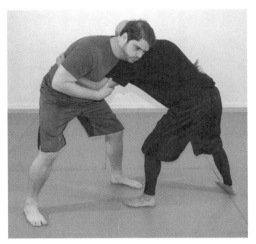 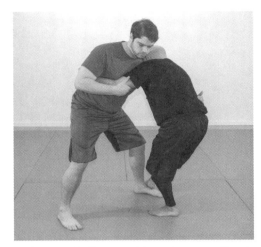

From the over-under clinch (left legs forward), Dave pulls. This makes Dave's front leg lighter.

Andrew capitalizes on this and sweeps Dave's front leg from right to left on the ankle with the sole of his right foot.

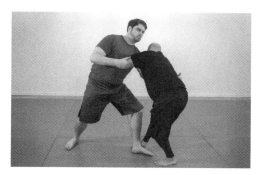

Andrew finishes the sweep by twisting with his upper body to the right so Dave hits the ground.

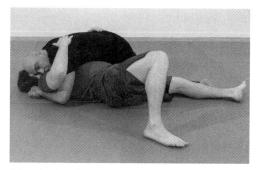

After Andrew's opponent hits the ground, he is sure to follow up immediately with ground techniques. If there is too much separation between Andrew and his opponent after grounding him, Andrew is probably going to lose the advantage.

Outside Leg Trip (Sotogake)

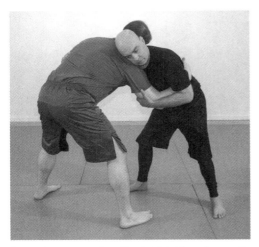 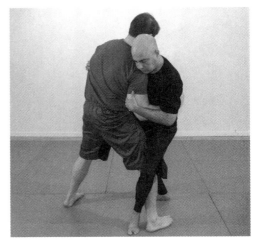

From the over-under clinch (right legs forward), Dave pulls.

Capitalizing on this, Andrew enters in fully with his rear (left) leg and entangles it deeply, from the outside, on Dave's front (right) leg.

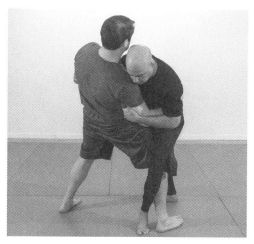

To finish the takedown, Andrew drives forward and leans in with his upper body while pulling the outside hooked leg and takes Dave down onto his back.

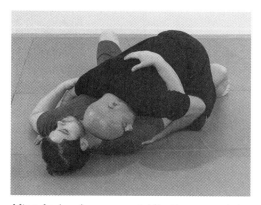

After Andrew's opponent hits the ground, he is sure to follow up immediately with ground techniques.

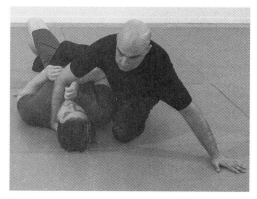

If there is too much separation between Andrew and his opponent after grounding him, Andrew is probably going to lose the advantage. The top MMA fighter Lyoto Machida has taken down many elite MMA fighters with this outside leg trip (sotogake).

Outside Thigh Scoop (Sotokomata)

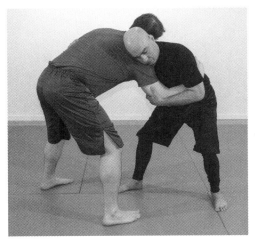

From the over-under clinch (right legs forward), Dave pulls Andrew, which makes Dave's front leg lighter.

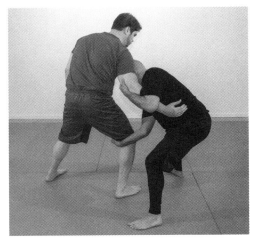

Andrew capitalizes on this by fully stepping in with his rear leg and lifting Dave's front leg from the outside with his disengaged right underhook arm.

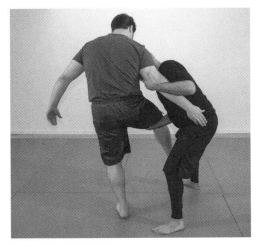

Andrew grips Dave's right arm tightly with his left overhook for control and buries his head and shoulder into Dave's shoulder and chest. When Andrew goes to take Dave's leg, he squats low so he uses his hips to elevate the leg, not just his arms. Dave is then driven onto his back.

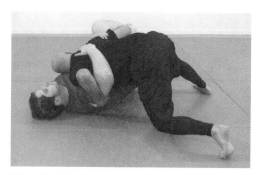

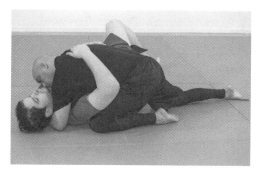

After Andrew's opponent hits the ground, he is sure to follow up immediately with ground techniques.

If there is too much separation between Andrew and his opponent after grounding him, Andrew is probably going to lose the advantage.

Rear Foot Sweep (Susoharai)

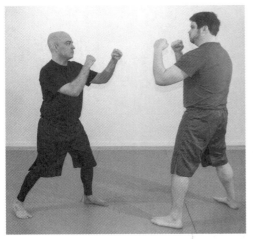

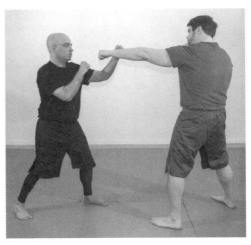

Andrew and Dave are facing each other in MMA fighting stances (left legs forward). Andrew performs an arm-pull force out (*hikkake*) attempt to place Dave into a perpendicular position.

Dave extends his left arm for an attack.

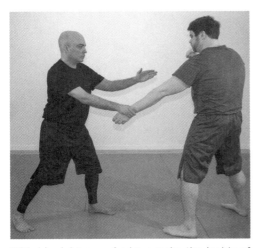

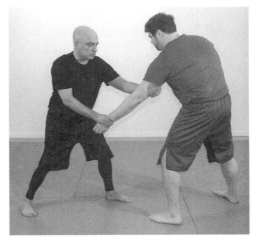

With his right arm, Andrew grabs the inside of Dave's left wrist and jerks it down low.

Then with his left hand, Andrew reaches under Dave's left arm to grab it by the triceps.

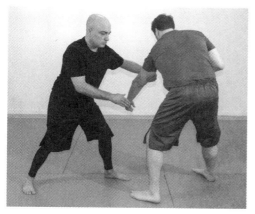

He pulls Dave's arm across his body. This places Dave into a perpendicular position when the move doesn't work.

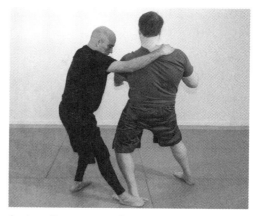

Andrew then sweeps Dave's front leg from the rear.

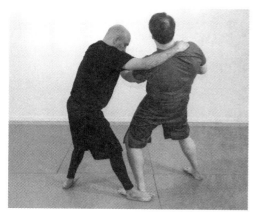

He finishes the sweep by using his upper body to pull Dave to the ground.

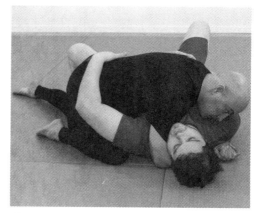

After Andrew's opponent hits the ground, he is sure to follow up immediately with ground techniques. If there is too much separation between Andrew and his opponent after grounding him, Andrew is probably going to lose the advantage.

Ankle Pick (Susotori)

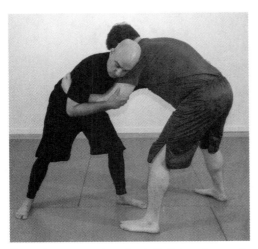 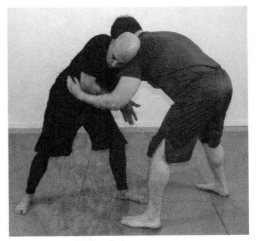

From the over-under clinch (left legs forward), Dave pulls Andrew, which makes Dave's front leg lighter.

Andrew swims his right overhook into a right underhook to get inside control.

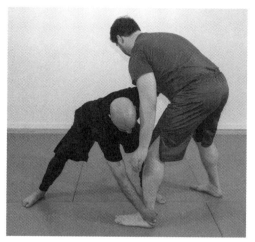

With his right hand Andrew reaches down and grabs Dave's left ankle.

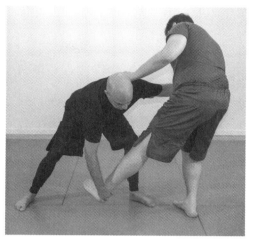

While Andrew elevates the grabbed ankle, he drives Dave onto his back as he also applies a left underhook.

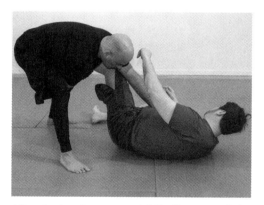

After Andrew's opponent hits the ground, he is sure to follow up immediately with ground techniques.

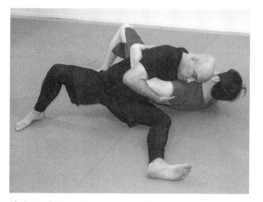

If there is too much separation between Andrew and his opponent after grounding him, Andrew is probably going to lose the advantage.

Inside Leg Trip (Uchigake)

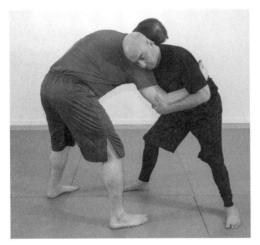

From the over-under clinch (right legs forward), Dave pulls.

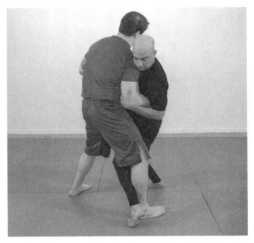

Capitalizing on this, Andrew enters in fully with his rear (left) leg and entangles it deeply, from the inside, with Dave's front (right) leg.

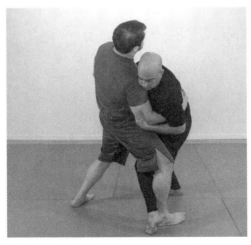

To finish the takedown, Andrew drives forward while pulling the inside hooked leg and takes Dave down onto his back.

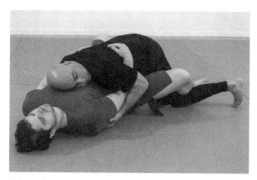

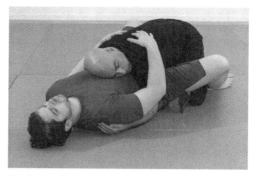

After Andrew's opponent hits the ground, he is sure to follow up immediately with ground techniques.

If there is too much separation between Andrew and his opponent after grounding him, Andrew is probably going to lose the advantage.

Thigh-Grabbing Push Down (Watashikomi)

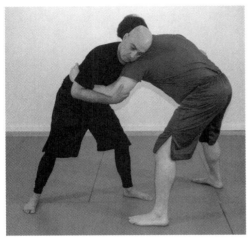

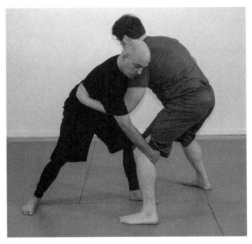

From the over-under clinch (left legs forward), Dave pulls Andrew, which makes Dave's front leg lighter.

Andrew reaches down with his right overhook arm and grabs Dave's front left leg at the hamstring or behind the knee.

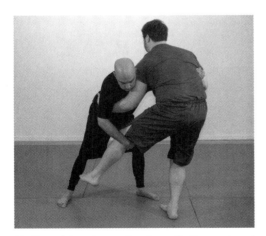

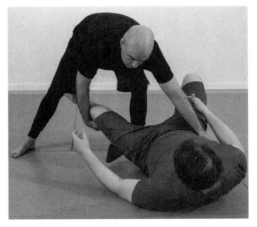

He then drives forward as he pulls the captured leg toward him, which will make Dave fall onto his back.

After Andrew's opponent hits the ground, he is sure to follow up immediately with ground techniques.

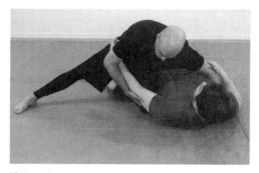 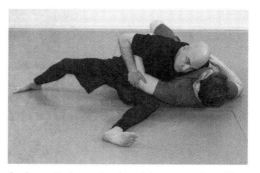

If there is too much separation between Andrew and his opponent after grounding him, Andrew is probably going to lose the advantage.

Andrew attains a dominant top ground position on Dave.

Twist-Down Techniques (Hinerite)

Kimarite twist-down techniques, as the name implies, involve you twisting your opponent in a circular manner to take him down. *Hineri* is the Japanese word for "twist." Usually with twisting techniques, your opponent is pushing into you to ideally affect the move. Many of these twisting takedowns control your opponent's upper body to ground him while several less common ones painfully lock out your opponent's elbow.

Fisherman's Throw (Amiuchi)

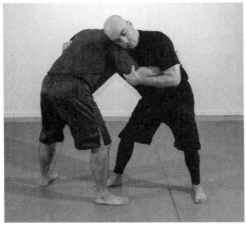

Andrew and Matt begin in the over-under clinch (right legs forward).

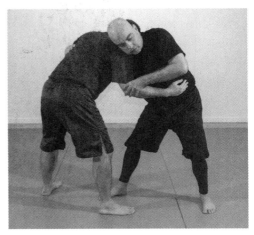

Andrew pushes Matt's underhook down at the elbow with his left overhook.

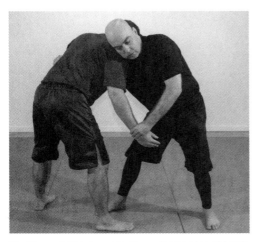

He then slides down to the wrist to clear Matt's underhook from his body.

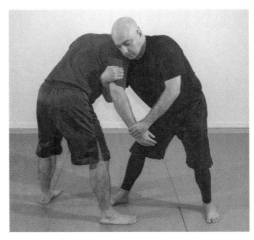

Andrew disengages his right underhook. He then quickly underhooks Matt's right arm at the triceps area.

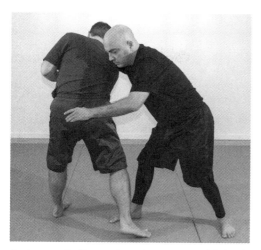

Andrew pulls the captured arm across his body with his right arm.

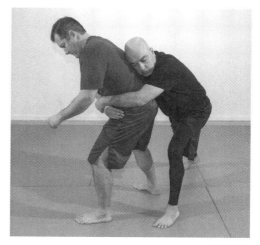

He can then achieve the rear clinch. This kimarite has been modified to suit the MMA fighter, but it is similar to how the Japanese traditionally throw a fishing net, hence the name.

Clasped-Hand Twist Down (Gasshohineri)

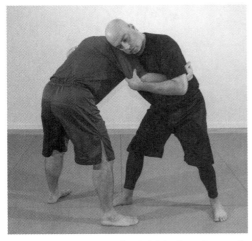

From the over-under clinch (right legs forward), Matt pushes.

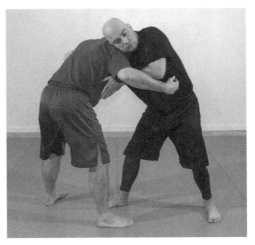

Andrew swims his left overhook into a left underhook.

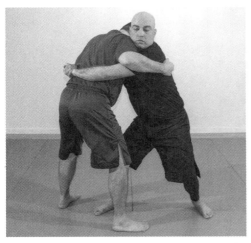

He then achieves double underhooks while clasping his hands together.

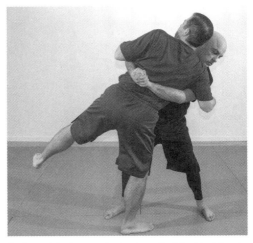

Going with the push, Andrew twists his hips to his left in order to toss Matt to the ground.

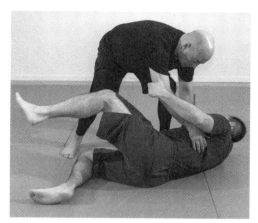

After Andrew's opponent hits the ground, he is sure to follow up immediately with ground techniques.

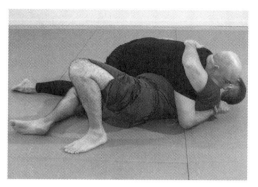

If there is too much separation between Andrew and his opponent after grounding him, Andrew is probably going to lose the advantage.

Two-Handed Arm Twist Down (Kainahineri)

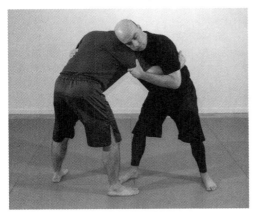

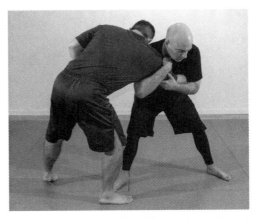

From the over-under clinch (right legs forward), Matt pushes in heavily.

Andrew disengages his right underhook and deeply underhooks Matt's underhook. Andrew goes with this push by first opening up his rear foot to the side.

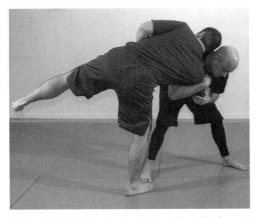

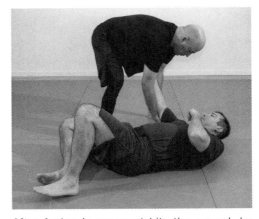

He twists his hips to the left while pivoting on his feet and strongly twists Matt's right arm until he hits the ground.

After Andrew's opponent hits the ground, he is sure to follow up immediately with ground techniques.

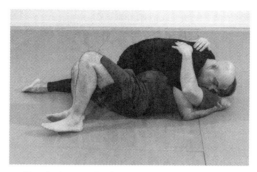

If there is too much separation between Andrew and his opponent after grounding him, Andrew is probably going to lose the advantage. With this twisting takedown, there is the danger of your opponent taking your back into the rear clinch if the takedown fails.

Under-Shoulder Swing Down (Katasukashi)

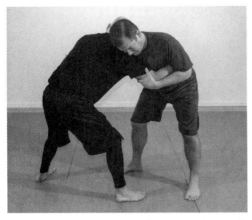

From the over-under clinch (right legs forward), Matt pushes.

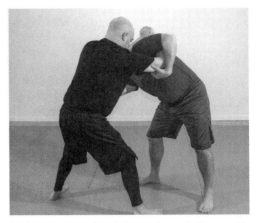

Andrew goes with this push and then pulls Matt's right shoulder down with a deep right underhook that is assisted by clasping his hands together in a palm-to-palm grip.

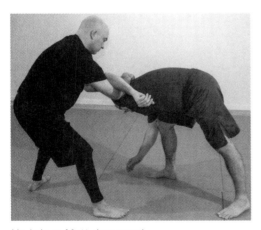

He brings Matt downward.

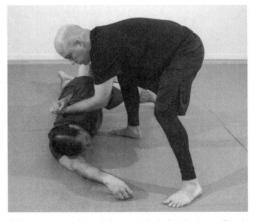

With a twist of his hips to his left, Andrew finalizes the takedown by backing away in order to throw Matt onto his stomach.

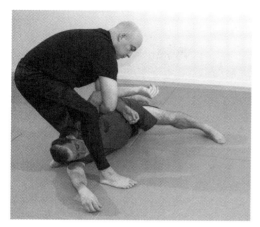

Andrew then spins into a BJJ–style armlock to finish him off.

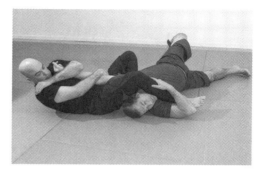

He pinches his knees together to control Matt's body and makes sure that Matt's hand is pointing thumb upward to properly lock the elbow. Matt's arm is trapped on Andrew's torso while Andrew elevates his hips to hyper-extend Matt's elbow. This kimarite flows nicely into an armlock.

Armlock Twist Down (Kotehineri)

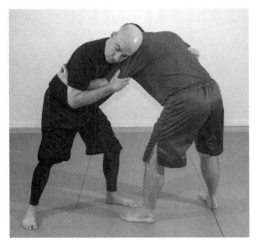

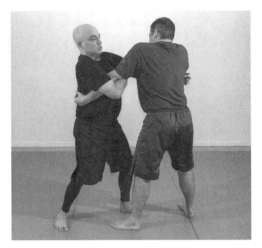

From the over-under clinch (left legs forward), Matt pushes.

Andrew elbow locks Matt's underhook from below by lifting his deeply sunk-in right over-hook. This elbow lock lifts Matt onto his toes and unbalances him.

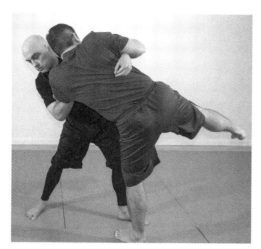

Capitalizing on this, Andrew first opens his rear foot to the side so he can turn his hips to the right by pivoting on his feet.

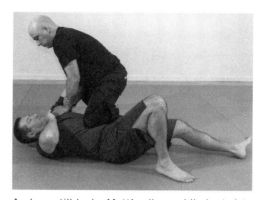

Andrew still locks Matt's elbow while he twists him to the ground. Andrew applies a BJJ–style elbow lock from the knee-on-belly position. This kimarite flows nicely into an elbow lock on the ground.

Head-Twisting Throw (Kubihineri)

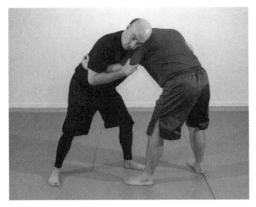

From the over-under clinch (left legs forward), Matt pushes.

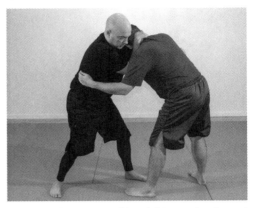

Andrew disengages his right overhook and secures a tight grip on Matt's neck.

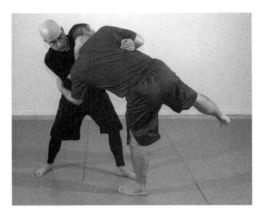

Andrew first opens his rear foot to the side so he can turn his hips to the right by pivoting on his feet. At the same time, Andrew twists Matt to the ground with the solid grip on Matt's neck and with the assistance of his left underhook.

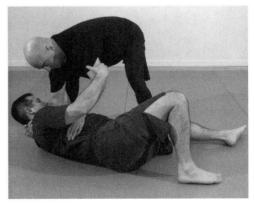

After Andrew's opponent hits the ground, he is sure to follow up immediately with ground techniques.

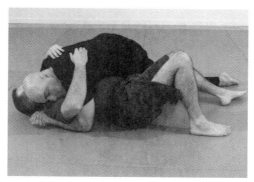

If there is too much separation between Andrew and his opponent after grounding him, Andrew is probably going to lose the advantage.

Twist Down (Makiotoshi)

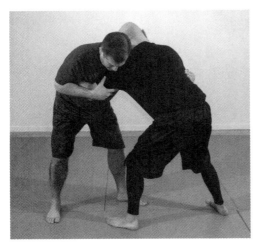

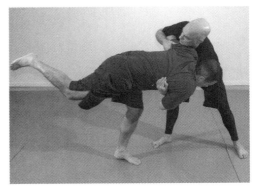

From the over-under clinch (left legs forward), Matt pushes.

Andrew, capitalizing on the push, steps back fully with his left leg while maintaining a tight upper body hold. As Andrew twists Matt downward to the ground, he pushes on Matt's arm with his right overhook arm and pulls with his left underhook to assist him.

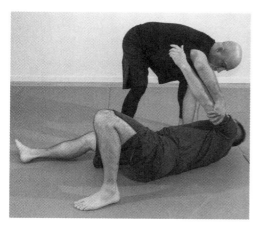

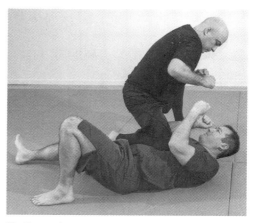

After Andrew's opponent hits the ground, he is sure to follow up immediately with ground techniques.

If there is too much separation between Andrew and his opponent after grounding him, Andrew is probably going to lose the advantage.

Outer-Thigh-Sweep Twist Down (Sotomuso)

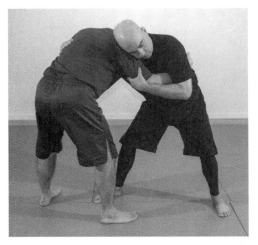

From the over-under clinch (right legs forward), Matt pushes.

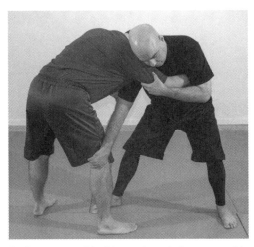

Andrew goes with this push and disengages his right underhook. Andrew quickly reaches across with his right hand to block Matt's front leg.

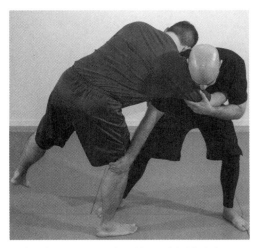

While tightly controlling Matt with his left over-hook and blocking Matt's front leg, Andrew twists his body to his left and thereby forces Matt to the ground.

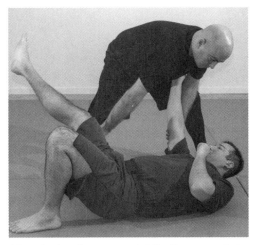

After Andrew's opponent hits the ground, he is sure to follow up immediately with ground techniques.

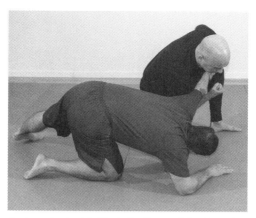

Using his whole body, Andrew locks Matt's left elbow while dropping down to his right knee to take Matt to the ground.

Armbar-Throw Counter (Sakatottari)

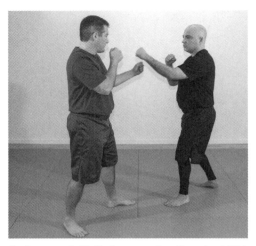

Andrew and Matt face each other in MMA fighting stances (left legs forward).

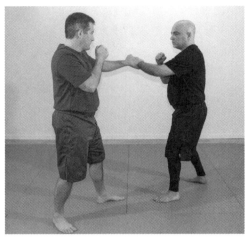

Matt grabs Andrew's left wrist with his left hand and jerks it down. Matt is attempting the armbar throw (tottari).

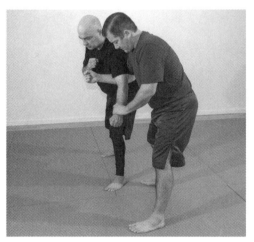

At the same time, Matt steps in to Andrew's left side with his right foot. As Matt steps fully in, he pulls Andrew's left arm across his body until Andrew's wrist is near Matt's left hip. Matt then pivots on his right foot, swinging his left leg behind him. When Matt pivots, he weaves his right arm so his inner mid-forearm area presses on the crook of Andrew's captured left elbow.

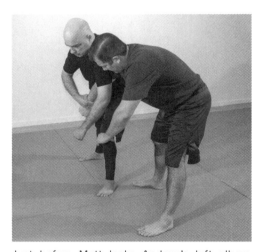

Just before Matt locks Andrew's left elbow, Andrew frees his left wrist from Matt's grip. In the same motion, Andrew grabs Matt's right wrist with his right hand and twists Matt's wrist so Matt's thumb is pointing down.

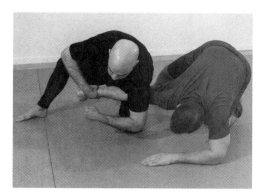

Andrew then uses his freed left arm to weave over Matt's captured right arm so his armpit is on Matt's right elbow. Using his whole body, Andrew locks Matt's right elbow while dropping down to his left knee to take Matt to the ground.

Thrust Down Forward (Tsukiotoshi)

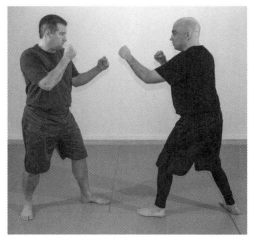

Andrew and Matt are facing each other in MMA fighting stances (left legs forward).

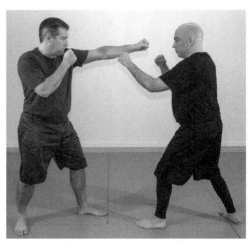

Matt extends his left arm in a committed attack.

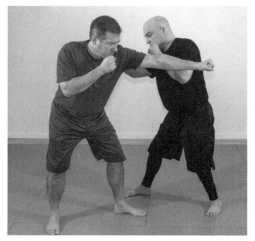

Andrew avoids this attack by fully stepping in with his right foot to Matt's left side. As Andrew steps in, he strongly slaps Matt's left shoulder blade with his right hand.

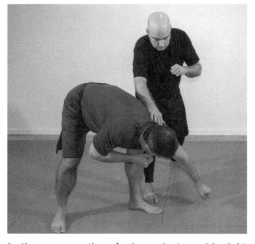

In the same motion, Andrew pivots on his right foot and swings his left leg behind him.

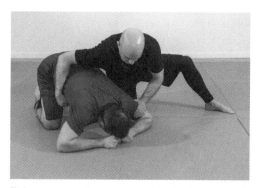

This sudden slap brings Matt to the ground. After Andrew's opponent hits the ground, he is sure to follow up immediately with ground techniques.

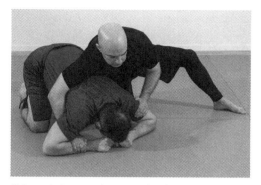

If there is too much separation between Andrew and his opponent after grounding him, Andrew is probably going to lose the advantage.

Inner-Thigh-Sweep Twist Down (Uchimuso)

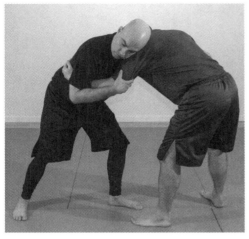

From the over-under clinch (left legs forward), Matt pulls Andrew, which makes Matt's front leg lighter.

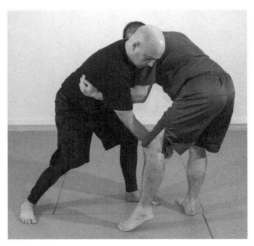

Andrew capitalizes on this pull and elevates Matt's front leg from the inside with his disengaged right overhook arm.

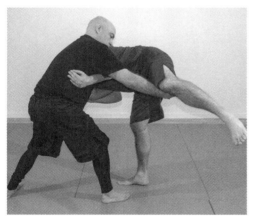

Andrew steps fully back with his left leg and twists his hips to the left by pivoting on his feet.

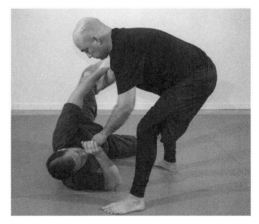

He then drives Matt onto his back by elevating Matt's left leg. After Andrew's opponent hits the ground, he is sure to follow up immediately with ground techniques.

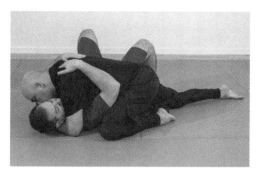

If there is too much separation between Andrew and his opponent after grounding him, Andrew is probably going to lose the advantage.

Head-Pivot Throw (Zubuneri)

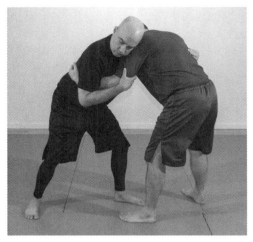

From the over-under clinch (left legs forward), Matt pushes Andrew.

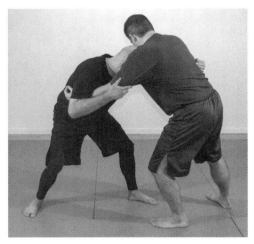

Capitalizing on this push, Andrew buries the top of his head into Matt's chest.

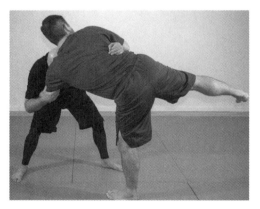

Andrew turns his hips to the right by pivoting on his feet, which causes Matt to fall.

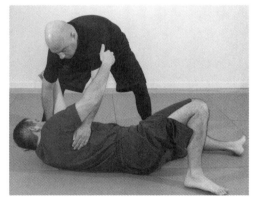

With Andrew's head still buried in Matt's chest, Andrew throws Matt to his right by using his head as a pivot point. After Andrew's opponent hits the ground, he is sure to follow up immediately with ground techniques.

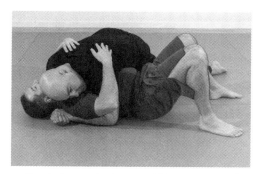

If there is too much separation between Andrew and his opponent after grounding him, Andrew is probably going to lose the advantage.

Special Techniques (Tokushuwaza)

Kimarite special techniques, as the name implies, are techniques that offer unique methods of taking down your opponent. Some take down your opponent from the rear clinch while others require you to pull your opponent to the ground from the front. For the kimarite that begin from the rear clinch, to first obtain the rear clinch, you would have to perform a kimarite like arm-grabbing force out (hikkake) or fisherman's throw (amiuchi), which are described in this book.

Slap Down (Hatakikomi)

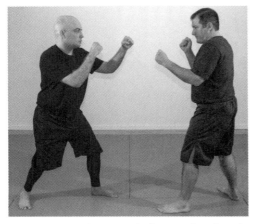 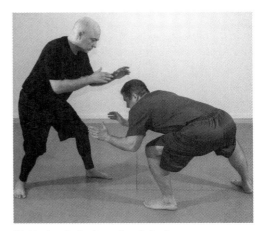

Andrew and Matt are facing each other in MMA fighting stances (left legs forward).

Matt shoots in for a low takedown.

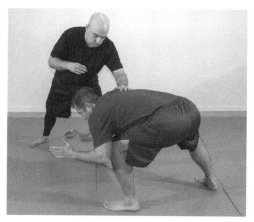

Andrew enters in strongly to his left. He slaps Matt on the shoulder or back to make Matt hit the ground.

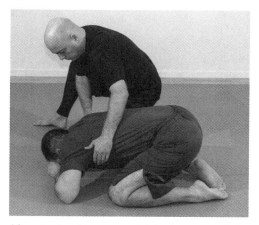

After Andrew's opponent hits the ground, he is sure to follow up immediately with ground techniques.

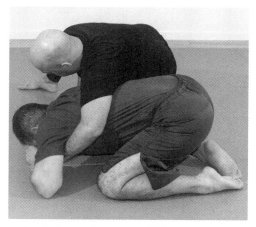

If there is too much separation between Andrew and his opponent after grounding him, Andrew is probably going to lose the advantage.

Hand Pull Down (Hikiotoshi)

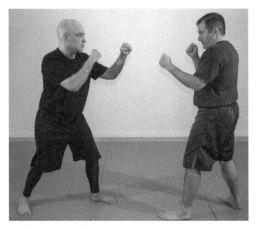

Andrew and Matt are facing each other in MMA fighting stances (left legs forward).

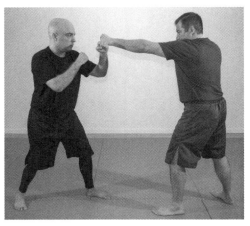

Matt extends his left arm for an attack.

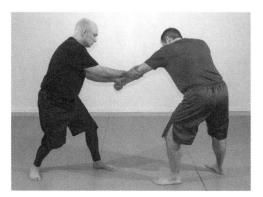

Andrew grabs Matt's arm with both of his arms and pulls Matt to the ground by moving Andrew's body backward.

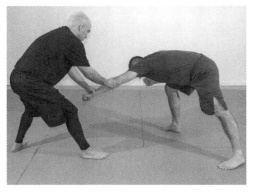

After Andrew's opponent hits the ground, he is sure to follow up immediately with ground techniques.

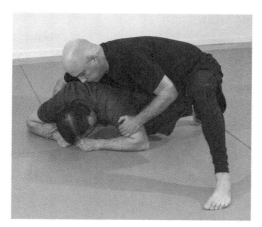

If there is too much separation between Andrew and his opponent after grounding him, Andrew is probably going to lose the advantage.

Arm-Pull Force Out (Hikkake)

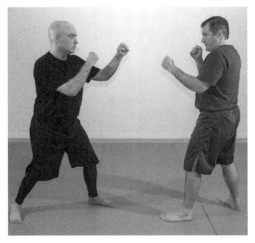

Andrew and Matt are facing each other in MMA fighting stances (left legs forward).

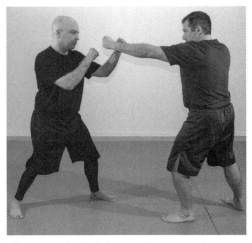

Matt extends his left arm for an attack.

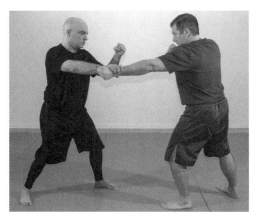

Andrew, with his right arm, grabs the inside of Matt's left wrist and jerks it down low.

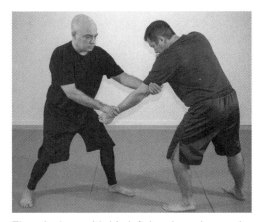

Then Andrew with his left hand reaches under Matt's left arm to grab it by the triceps.

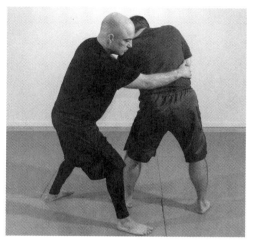

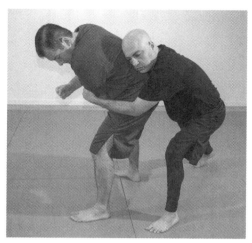

He pulls Matt's left arm across his body with his left arm, while taking Matt's back with his right arm.

He then attains the rear clinch on Matt.

Armbar Force Down (Kimetaoshi)

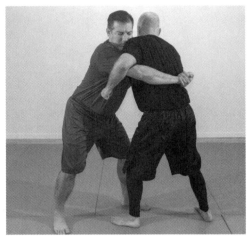

Matt has Andrew in the double-underhooks clinch (left legs forward).

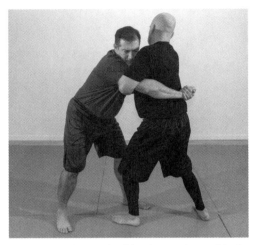

Andrew reaches under Matt's armpits and locks his hands together palm to palm, achieving the kannuki hold.

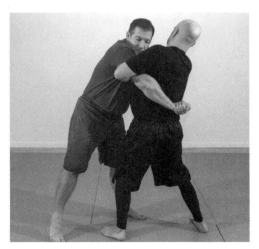

Andrew lifts Matt up with his kannuki hold to break his balance.

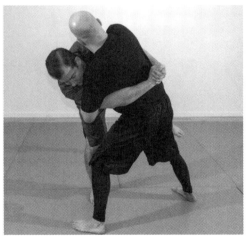

To finish, Andrew throws Matt down by shuffling forward with his hips and legs.

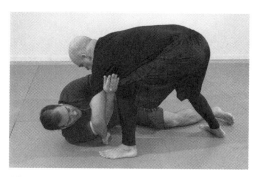

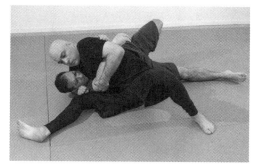

After Andrew's opponent hits the ground, he is sure to follow up immediately with ground techniques.

If there is too much separation between Andrew and his opponent after grounding him, Andrew is probably going to lose the advantage.

Rear Leg Trip (Okurigake)

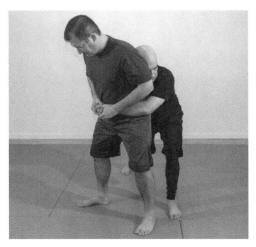

Andrew has Matt in the rear clinch.

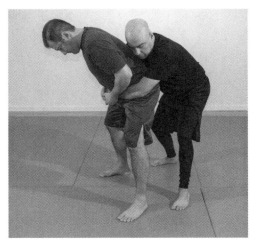

Matt begins to walk forward trying to escape.

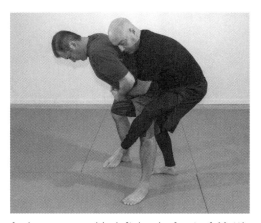

Andrew weaves his left leg in front of Matt's left leg above his knee.

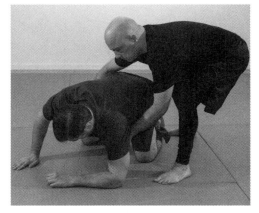

This leg trip with Matt's forward momentum causes him to fall on his left side. After Andrew's opponent hits the ground, he is sure to follow up immediately with ground techniques.

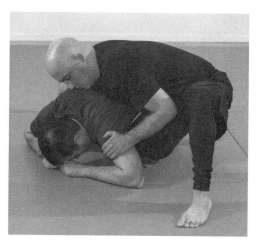

If there is too much separation between Andrew and his opponent after grounding him, Andrew is probably going to lose the advantage.

Rear Pull Down (Okurihikiotoshi)

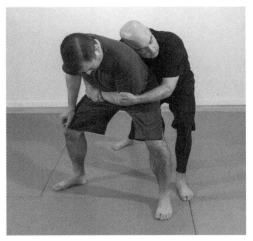 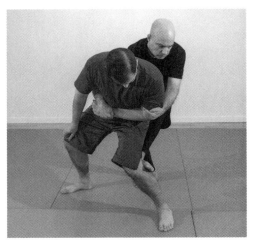

Andrew has Matt in the rear clinch with a two-on-one hold on Matt's left arm. Matt sinks his base down by squatting with his legs.

Andrew with the sole of his left foot presses on the back of Matt's left knee to break his balance. As Andrew presses in with his left foot, he sinks his right leg down for balance and presses with his left hip into his left foot for more pressure.

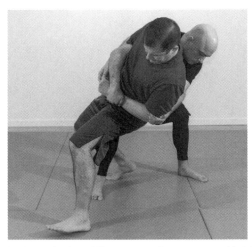

After Matt's balance is broken, Andrew disengages the press on Matt's knee and steps back fully with his left leg.

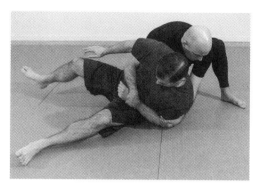 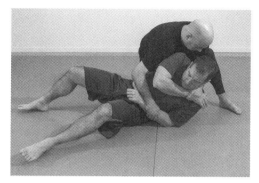

Andrew pulls Matt down to the ground by turning his hips to the left by pivoting on his feet.

After Matt hits the ground, Andrew follows up by wrapping Matt's right arm around his neck to secure a dominant ground position. After Andrew's opponent hits the ground, he is sure to follow up immediately with ground techniques. If there is too much separation between Andrew and his opponent after grounding him, Andrew is probably going to lose the advantage.

Rear Throw Down (Okurinage)

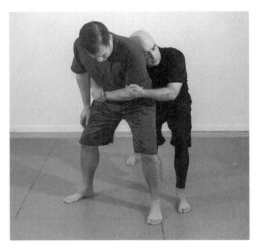 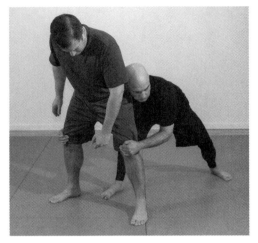

Andrew has Matt in the rear clinch with a two-on-one hold on Matt's left arm.

Andrew releases the rear clinch and then slides his hands down in front of Matt's knees. Andrew then places his right shoulder on Matt's buttocks. Lowering his level, Andrew's right leg is forward bending at the knee with his left leg behind pressing in.

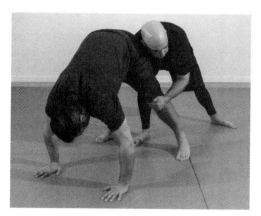

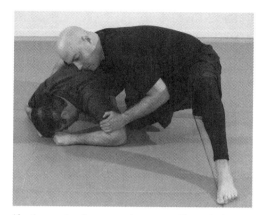

He pulls with his hands on the knees and drives forward with his legs and torso to make Matt fall forward hard on the ground. After Andrew's opponent hits the ground, he is sure to follow up immediately with ground techniques.

If there is too much separation between Andrew and his opponent after grounding him, Andrew is probably going to lose the advantage.

Rear-Lift Body Slam (Okuritsuriotoshi)

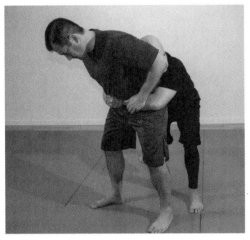

Andrew has Matt in the rear clinch.

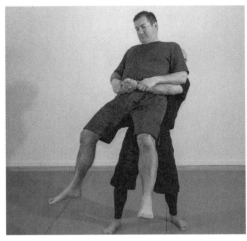

While tightly maintaining his rear clinch, Andrew lifts Matt into the air using his hips and legs.

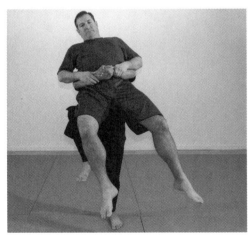

While Matt is airborne, Andrew lifts his bent right leg high and then quickly moves it sideways across Matt's right knee.

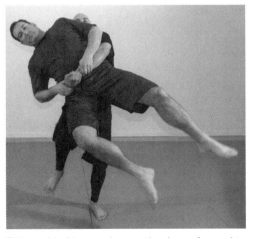

This rapid sideways leg motion is performed to rotate Matt's body so that when Andrew drops Matt, he will land on all fours and not end up back on his feet.

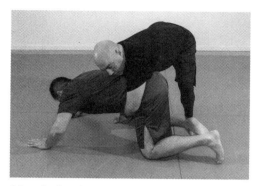

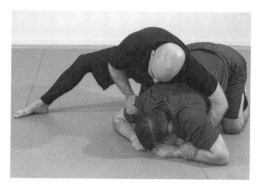

After Andrew's opponent hits the ground, he is sure to follow up immediately with ground techniques.

If there is too much separation between Andrew and his opponent after grounding him, Andrew is probably going to lose the advantage.

Head Slap Down (Sokubiotoshi)

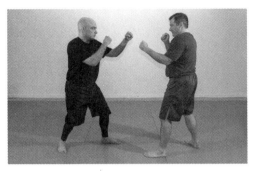

Andrew and Matt are facing each other in MMA fighting stances (left legs forward).

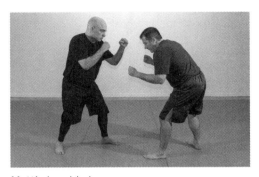

Matt's head is low.

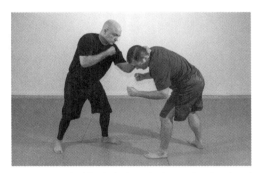

Andrew with his left hand slaps the back of Matt's head down, lowering his head and torso.

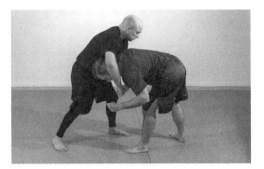

With his right arm, Andrew sinks in a BJJ–style guillotine choke to finish Matt off.

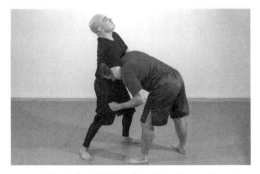

This sumo technique was modified for MMA after the head slap down to include a finishing hold, the guillotine choke.

Conclusion

Sumo is the fusion of honored ritual with unbridled power. Even in a combat sport like sumo, where great body mass and girth are often winning factors, superior technique can overcome size and strength. Some of these sumo techniques may look familiar to many grapplers, because there are only so many ways you can take someone down, and many popular grappling arts are derived from the same source: jujitsu.

"Sumo is the primogenitor of all martial arts and ways that came later in Japan. When we practice our *budo* (Japanese martial ways) today, in some ways we are carrying on an ancient tradition, tapping into a current that electrifies our training and lifts it into a sphere far beyond that of other activities."[44]

Nonetheless, looking at takedowns and throws from a sumo perspective can give you a great advantage in your MMA grappling game. Other martial artists, especially competitive grapplers like judo, sambo, and Brazilian jiu-jitsu practitioners, can benefit technically from the knowledge and application of sumo techniques. Of course, to really gain the full potential of sumo techniques, the training of the techniques should be done in live-grappling sparring, after the basic mechanics of the techniques are thoroughly drilled. Perhaps, after reading this book, you may become inspired to add a few sumo techniques to your own martial arts arsenal. A dynamic sumo move may just be another piece of the puzzle in your quest for more effective fighting techniques. Sumo, the root of jujitsu, has much to offer all martial artists.

Bibliography

Buckingham, Dorothea N. *The Essential Guide to Sumo*. Honolulu, HI: The Bess Press, 1994.

Draeger, Donn F. and Robert W. Smith. *Asian Fighting Arts*. New York: Berkley Medallion Books, 1969.

Funakoshi, Gichin. *Karate-Do, My Way of Life*. New York: Kodansha International, 1975.

Gladwell, Malcolm. *David and Goliath: Underdogs, Misfits, and the Art of Battling Giants*. New York: Little, Brown and Company, 2013.

Gracie, Renzo and John Danaher. *Mastering Jujitsu*. Champaign, IL: Human Kinetics, 2003.

Hall, Mina. *The Big Book of Sumo*. Berkeley CA: Stone Bridge Press, 1997.

Japan Travel Bureau. *Illustrated Martial Arts and Sports in Japan*. Tokyo: Japan Travel Bureau, 1993.

Kawamura, Teizo and Toshiro Daigo. *Kodokan New Japanese-English Dictionary of Judo*. Tokyo: The Foundation of Kodokan Judo Institute, 2000.

Kubota, Makoto. *Sumo*. San Francisco, CA: Chronicle Books, 1996.

Lowry, Dave. "Sumo: The Oldest Budo." *Black Belt*, February 1992, 92. https://books.google.com.

Machida, Lyoto, Glen Cordoza, and Erich Krauss. *Machida Karate-Do Mixed Martial Arts Techniques*. Auberry, CA: Victory Belt Publishing, 2009.

Misawa, Masatoshi. *Sumo's Winning Ways: The Enigma of the 82 Kimarite,* video. Tokyo: Japan Broadcasting Corporation, 2006.

Newton, Clyde. *Dynamic Sumo*. New York: Kodansha International, 1994

Ozkaptan, Halim, Crosbie E. Saint, and Robert S. Fiero. *Conquering Fear: Development of Courage in Soldiers and Other High-Risk Occupations*. Raleigh, NC: Lulu Press, 2007.

Pearlstein, Ferne. *Sumo East and West*, video. United States: SumoFilms Inc., 2003.

Peligro, Kid. *The Gracie Way*. Montpelier, VT: Invisible Cities Press, 2003.

Reid, T. R. "Sumo." *National Geographic* 192, no. 1 (1997): 42–57.

Sackett, Joel and Wes Benson. *Rikishi: The Men of Sumo*. Tokyo: John Weatherhill, 1986.

Stevens, John. *Abundant Peace: The Biography of Morihei Ueshiba, Founder of Aikido*. Boston: Shambhala Publications, 1987.

———. *The Way of Judo: A Portrait of Jigoro Kano & His Students*. Boston: Shambhala Publications, 2013.

———. *Three Budo Masters*. Tokyo: Kodansha International, 1995.

Tuckett, Phil. *Sports Illustrated's Get the Feeling: POWER!*, video. New York: HBO Video, 1988.

Uyenishi, Sada Kazu. *The Text-Book of Ju-Jutsu as Practised in Japan*. Thousand Oaks, CA: Dragon Associates, Inc., 1997.

Zabel, Thomas. *Sumo Skills, Instructional Guide for Competitive Sumo*. Mico, TX: Ozumo Academy Publishing, 2014.

-

Notes

Chapter 1: Sumo Wrestling Overview

1. Renzo Gracie and John Danaher, *Mastering Jujitsu* (Champaign, IL: Human Kinetics, 2003), 8–11.

2. In this book we will follow the modern convention of using "jujitsu" when describing the Japanese style and "jiu-jitsu" when discussing the Brazilian style. However, some older sources referenced herein may use the "jiu jitsu" or "jujutsu" spelling for the Japanese style. In any case, all of the spelling variations for this word basically mean the same thing.

3. Donn F. Draeger and Robert W. Smith, *Asian Fighting Arts* (New York: Berkley Medallion Books, 1969), 138.

4. John Stevens, *The Way of Judo: Portrait of Jigoro Kano and His Students* (Boston: Shambhala Publications, 2013), 9, 17.

5. Gichin Funakoshi, *Karate-Do, My Way of Life* (New York: Kodansha International, 1975), 122–124.

6. John Stevens, *Abundant Peace: The Biography of Morihei Ueshiba, Founder of Aikido* (Boston: Shambhala Publications, 1987), 67–68.

7. John Stevens, *Three Budo Masters* (Tokyo: Kodansha International, 1995), 7.

8. Lyoto Machida, Glen Cordoza, and Erich Krauss, *Machida Karate-Do Mixed Martial Arts Techniques* (Auberry, CA: Victory Belt Publishing, 2009), 11–13, 15, 124, 148–149.

9. Mina Hall, *The Big Book of Sumo* (Berkeley, CA: Stone Bridge Press, 1997), 21.

10. Ferne Pearlstein, *Sumo East and West* (United States: SumoFilms Inc., 2003), video.

11. Masatoshi Misawa, *Sumo's Winning Ways: The Enigma of the 82 Kimarite* (Tokyo: Japan Broadcasting Corporation, 2006), video.

Chapter 2: Sumo Wrestling Case Studies

12. Ibid.

13. Ibid.

14. Pearlstein, *Sumo East and West.*

15. T. R. Reid, "Sumo," *National Geographic* 192, no. 1 (1997): 42–57.

16. Pearlstein, *Sumo East and West.*

17. Hall, *The Big Book of Sumo,* 126.

18. Pearlstein, *Sumo East and West.*

19. Phil Tuckett, *Sports Illustrated's Get the Feeling: POWER!* (New York: HBO Video, 1988), video.

20. Misawa, *Sumo's Winning Ways.*

21. Stevens, *Three Budo Masters,* 69.

22. Thomas Zabel, *Sumo Skills, Instructional Guide for Competitive Sumo* (Mico, TX: Ozumo Academy Publishing, 2014), 31.

23. Ibid., 31, 45.

24. Dorothea N. Buckingham, *The Essential Guide to Sumo* (Honolulu, HI: The Bess Press, 1994), 142–143.

25. Pearlstein, *Sumo East and West.*

26. Misawa, *Sumo's Winning Ways.*

27. Ibid.

28. Teizo Kawamura and Toshiro Daigo, *Kodokan New Japanese-English Dictionary of Judo* (Tokyo: The Foundation of Kodokan Judo Institute, 2000), 133.

29. Misawa, *Sumo's Winning Ways.*

Chapter 3: Sumo and MMA

30. Gracie and Danaher, *Mastering Jujitsu*, 95.

31. Ibid., 149.

32. Stevens, *The Way of Judo,* 141–142.

33. Machida, Cordoza, and Krauss, *Machida Karate-Do Mixed Martial Arts Techniques*, 11–12.

34. Ibid., 124.

35. Ibid., 148–149.

36. Ibid., 13.

37. Ibid., 15.

38. Sada Kazu Uyenishi, *The Text-Book of Ju-Jutsu as Practised in Japan* (Thousand Oaks, CA: Dragon Associates, 1997), 3.

39. Kid Peligro, *The Gracie Way* (Montpelier, VT: Invisible Cities Press, 2003), 15–17.

40. Gracie and Danaher, *Mastering Jujitsu,* 203.

41. Halim Ozkaptan, Crosbie E. Saint, and Robert S. Fiero, *Conquering Fear: Development of Courage in Soldiers and Other High-Risk Occupations* (Raleigh, NC: Lulu Press, 2007).

42. Alexander the Great had many physicians. The source of the quote is unknown. Alexander the Great (Alexander III of Macedon) was king of the Ancient Greek kingdom of Macedon. He lived between July 356 BC and June 323 BC.

Chapter 4: Technical Photos

43. Gracie and Danaher, *Mastering Jujitsu,* 66.

44. Dave Lowry, "Sumo: The Oldest Budo," *Black Belt*, February 1992, 92. https://books .google.com.

Index

Abundant Peace (Stevens), 2, 155–156
aikido, 2, 155
Akebono (Chad George Haheo Rowan), 8, 14–17, 19, 90
Alexander the Great, 41, 156
Alexander the Great's chief physician, 41
amateur sumo, 9, 33
American football, 11
ancient records, 11
ankle pick (susotori), 22; in techniques, 100
ankle-sweep twist down (nimaigeri), 92
arm bar force down (kimetaoshi), 22; in techniques, 140
arm bar throw (tottari), 25; in techniques, 124, 126
arm bar throw counter (sakatottari), 25; in techniques, 126
arm pull force out (hikkake), 98, 134, 138
armlock, 25; in techniques, 72, 113–114
armlock throw (kotenage), 25; in techniques, 72
armlock twist down (kotehineri), 114

Bader, Ryan, 36
balance, 16–17, 19–20, 22, 27, 31–32, 35, 38, 41
balance breaking (kuzushi), 22, 35
Belém, Brazil, 35
Belgium, 34
beltless arm throw (sukuinage), 78
big toe, 20
BJJ practitioner, 32, 39
body-drop throw (nichonage), 76
body-to-body sensitivity, 35
boxing, 17, 19, 25–26, 32, 34, 40
boxing ring, 25, 34
Brazil, xv, xvii, 2, 33–35, 38, 151, 155, 157
Brazilian jiu-jitsu (BJJ), xv, xvii, 2, 32–36, 38–39, 57–59, 73, 113, 115, 150–151, 157
breakfalls (ukemi), 5; in techniques, 43–51
budo, 151, 155–156

cage, 25, 30
chanko-nabe, 6
China, 3–4
clasped-hand twist down (gasshohineri), 108

clinch, xv, xvii, 17, 22–23, 26–36, 39, 41; in techniques, 43, 53–60, 68, 70–72, 74, 76, 78, 80, 82, 84–88, 90, 92, 94, 96, 100, 102, 104, 106–108, 110–112, 114, 116, 118, 120–122, 130, 132, 134, 139–140, 142, 144, 146, 148, 157
clinch phase, 26, 30–32, 34, 39, 41, 53, 60
clinches, xv, xvii, 26–27, 32–33, 157
clinching, xv, 17, 26, 31–35, 39, 60
collar-and-elbow clinch, 28
combat sports, xiii, xvii, 26–28, 41
Conde Koma, 34
conquer fear, 41
Conquering Fear (Ozkaptan, Saint, and Fiero), 41, 156
core stability and sensitivity, 41
Couture, Randy, 36
cross-training, 31–32
Cuba, 34

Danaher, John, 27, 29, 41, 51, 155–156
David and Goliath, 25, 37
David and Goliath: Underdogs, Misfits, and the Art of Battling Giants (Gladwell), 37
deceiving the cat (nekodamashi), 14
Department Store of Techniques (Waza no Depaato), 13, 38, 60
disqualification, 5
dohyo, 1, 5, 9, 12, 16, 18–19
dohyo-iri (ring-entering ceremony), 16, 18
dominant clinch, 28–29
double-underhooks clinch, 22–23, 28–29; in techniques, 55, 58–59, 86–87, 140
driving power, 41

Edo period (AD 1603–1867), 4, 10
endurance, 41
Evans, Rashad, 36
explosiveness, 5, 12, 41

favorite techniques (tokui waza), 60
Fiero, Colonel Robert S., 41, 156
fighting spirit, 13, 34, 40
fisherman's throw (amiuchi), 106, 134

flexibility, 5, 12, 41
folkstyle, 11, 28, 32–33
football pass blocker, 17
former UFC Light Heavyweight Champion, 2, 37
forms (kata), 2, 8–9, 16, 98, 112
fortitude, 41
forty-eight hands (shijuuhatte), 10
forward breakfall (mae ukemi), 44–45
forward breakfall (mae ukemi) kneeling, 44
forward breakfall (mae ukemi) standing, 45
forward rolling breakfall (mae mawari ukemi),
    50–51
forward rolling breakfall (mae mawari ukemi)
    kneeling, 50
forward rolling breakfall (mae mawari ukemi)
    standing, 51
frame push escape, 59
France, 34
Franklin, Rich, 35–36
free-movement phase, 25–26, 30–32, 34, 51, 57, 60
front push down (oshitaoshi), 62, 66
front push out (oshidashi), 61, 64
front thrust down (tsukitaoshi), 62, 66
front thrust out (tsukidashi), 61, 64
fulcrum, 38
full hip throw (o-goshi), 2, 4
full shoulder throw (ippon seoi nage), 2, 4
Funakoshi, Gichin, 2–3, 19, 155

Gagamaru, 21
Gladwell, Malcolm, 37, 39
gloves, 19, 32
Gordeau, Gerard, 32
Gracie family, 33–35
Gracie, Carlos, 27, 29, 32–35, 38–39, 41, 51, 155–157
Gracie, Helio, 27, 29, 32–35, 38–39, 41, 51, 155–157
Gracie, Renzo, 27, 29, 32–35, 38–39, 41, 51, 155–157
Gracie, Royce, 27, 29, 32–35, 38–39, 41, 51, 155–157
grand champion (yokozuna), 8–9, 16–17
Grand Sumo Tournaments, 23
grappling, xv, xvii, 1, 11, 20, 28, 43, 56, 151, 157
Greco-Roman, 11, 28, 32
grip (yori), 10, 14, 16, 20, 22, 25–26, 28, 30–31, 41;
    in techniques, 53, 60, 88, 96, 112, 116, 122–123,
    126
gripping and pulling conditioning, 41
gripping strength, 41

grips, 26, 30–31; in techniques, 53, 88, 96
ground and pound, 33, 39, 42
ground fighting, 25–26, 29–33
ground phase, 26, 29–32, 34, 36, 39, 41, 43, 60
guard, 29, 33, 36, 39
guillotine choke, 73, 150

hand pull down (*hikiotoshi*), 136
hard principles, 38
harite (head slap), 20, 150
head pivot throw (zubuneri), 132
head slap down (sokubiotoshi), 150
head-twisting throw (kubihineri), 116
headhunting strikes, 51
headlock throw (kubinage), 74
Henderson, Dan, 36
hierarchy, 8
hinge, 26, 34, 39
hip throw (koshinage), 2, 4, 38; in techniques,
    71
hooking inner thigh throw (kakenage), 70

Imperial Army, 2
inner-thigh-lift throw (yaguranage), 80
inner thigh sweep twist down (*uchimuso*), 35;
    in techniques, 130
inside control, 22–23; in techniques, 53, 55, 60,
    82, 100
inside foot sweep (kekaeshi), 85
inside leg trip (uchigake), 15; in techniques, 102
inside thigh scoop (komatasukui), 88
Iron Man (Tetsujin), 18

Japan Sumo Association, 5, 10, 27, 60
Japan Sumo Association training school, 5
Japanese colony, 35
Japanese islands, 4
Japanese martial arts, 2, 5, 8, 21, 43
Japanese myth
Japanese schools, 9
Jimmerson, Art, 32
jiu-jitsu, xv, xvii, 2, 33–35, 38, 151, 155, 157
Jordan, Michael, 16
judo, xiii, xv, xvii, 1–2, 4, 8, 13, 21, 33–36, 38, 151,
    155–156
jujitsu, xiii, 1–2, 4, 12, 34, 38, 151, 155–156
jujutsu, 34, 155

K-1/Hero's 1 event, 36
Kakuryu, 16
kannuki hold, 22; in techniques, 140
Kano, Jigoro, 2–3, 21, 155
karate, xv, 2, 8, 19, 35–36, 155–156
Karate-Do, My Way of Life (Funakoshi), 2, 35, 155–156
kickboxer, 32
kimarite, 1, 4, 10–13, 15, 19, 22–23, 25, 27, 36, 38; in techniques, 43, 53, 60, 68, 73, 82, 90, 106–107, 113, 115, 134, 155
Kisenosato, 21
Kodokan Judo Institute, 34, 156
Kodokan New Japanese-English Dictionary of Judo (Kawamura and Daigo), 21, 156
komusubi, 13
Konishiki (Saleva'a Fuauli Atisano'e), 17–19
Korea, 4, 11
Korean wrestling (ssireum), 11

LeBell, Gene, 39
leg conditioning, 41
leg pick (ashitori), 11, 22; in techniques, 82
leg-tripping techniques (kakete), 38, 82
leverage, 14, 20, 22, 38, 58
live-grappling sparring, 151

Machida Karate-Do Mixed Martial Arts Techniques (Machida, Cordoza), 2, 35, 155–156
Machida, Lyoto "The Dragon", 2–3, 32, 35–37, 39, 42, 95, 155–156
Maeda, Mitsuyo "Count Trouble", 33–35
Mainoumi, 8, 13–15, 19, 22–23, 38, 60, 90
makiwara, 19
mawashi, 14, 16, 20
Meat Bomb, 17
medieval Japanese era, 10
Mexico, 34
mind-body connection, 41
mixed martial artist, xv, 40
MMA competitions, 25–26, 31
MMA fighters, 3, 8, 29–32, 37, 39, 51, 95
MMA fighting stance, 51–52, 61–62, 64, 66, 98, 124, 126, 128, 134, 136, 138, 150
MMA perspective, xvii, 12, 41–43
Mongolian grappling, 11
muay Thai, 32, 36
Myogiryu, 21

National Geographic, 16, 155
neutral clinch, 28
neutral position, 27
no-gi-cloth-required takedowns, 33
nodowa, 20

official tournament, 8
Okinawa, 2
Okinawan karate masters, 2
Okinawan sumo, 2
one-arm shoulder throw (ipponzeoi), 2, 4; in techniques, 68
one-dimensional striker, 39
Onishiki, 7, 17–19
open-hand attacks, 19–21, 34
Ortiz, Tito, 36
outer-thigh sweep twist down (sotomuso), 120
outside leg trip (sotogake), 2, 36; in techniques, 94–95
outside thigh scoop (sotokomata), 96
overarm (uwate), 27
overhook, 27; in techniques, 55–57, 60, 72, 75, 82, 86, 88, 90, 96, 100, 104, 106, 108, 114, 116, 118, 120, 122, 130
over-under clinch, 27–29, 35, 41; in techniques, 54–57, 68, 70–72, 74, 76, 78, 80, 82, 84–88, 90, 92, 94, 96, 100, 102, 104, 106, 108, 110, 112, 114, 116, 118, 120, 122, 130, 132
over-under clinch exercise, 56
Ozkaptan, Halim PhD, 41, 156

palm-to-palm grip, 53, 112
palms push escape, 58
Peligro, Kid, 38, 156
Penn, B. J., 36
phases of fighting, 32, 60
physical conditioning, 40–42
physical fitness, 41
physique, xvii, 6–7, 33
Portugal, 34
professional rikishi, 8, 13, 40
professional sumo, xiii, xvii, 8–9, 18–20
prohibited techniques, 5
psychological attitude, 40
psychological will, 41
pulling guard, 33
pulling heel hook (chongake), 84

push (oshi), xv, 2–7, 10, 13–14, 16–17, 19–22, 25, 27, 32, 34, 38–39; in techniques, 57–62, 64–72, 74, 76, 78, 80, 104, 106, 108, 110, 112, 114, 116, 118, 120, 122, 128, 132, 136, 140, 144, 148, 150, 155–156
push escape from the double-underhooks clinch, 58
push escape from the over-under clinch, 57
pushing sumo wrestling, 13

rank, 8–9, 13, 16–17, 19, 23, 35–36
rear breakfall (ushiro ukemi), 46–47
rear breakfall (ushiro ukemi) squatting, 46
rear breakfall (ushiro ukemi) standing, 47
rear clinch, 107, 111, 121, 134, 139, 142, 144, 146, 148
rear foot sweep (susoharai), 98
rear leg trip (okurigake), 142
rear lift body slam (okuritsuriotoshi), 148
rear lift out (okuritsuridashi), 11
rear pull down (okurihikiotoshi), 144
rear throw down (okurinage), 146
recipe for disaster, 32
riddle of the over-under clinch, 28
rikishi, 1, 5–23, 25, 28, 33, 38–40, 60, 73
ronin, 5–6
root of jujitsu, 1–2, 12, 38, 151
ryo-shitate, 22–23

s-grip, 53
Saint, General Crosbie E., 41, 156
sambo, xiii, xv, 151
samurai, 5–6, 10
samurai topknot hairstyle, 10
savate, 34
sekiwake, 19
self-defense, xvii, 2, 25, 33, 39
Severn, Dan, 39
shiko (foot stomping), 12, 104
Shotokan karate, 2, 35–36
shoulder-wheel throw (kata-guruma), 2
side breakfall (yoko ukemi), 48–49
side breakfall (yoko ukemi) lying down, 48
side breakfall (yoko ukemi) standing, 49
single and double legs, 33
slap, 10, 19–20, 25, 32, 34; in techniques, 44–51, 85, 128–129, 134–135, 150
slap down (hatakikomi), 19; in techniques, 134, 150

small outer hook (kosoto-gake), 2
social status, 8
soft principles, 38
South America, 34
southpaw, 36
Spain, 34
special techniques (tokushuwaza), 39, 134
sprawl and brawl, 32, 36, 39, 42
stablemaster, 5, 11, 21
Stablemaster Naruto (Takanosato), 21
Stablemaster Oyama, 11
street fights, 30
strength, 2, 5, 9, 13–14, 16–17, 19, 23, 25, 27, 30, 37–41, 151
strikes, 20, 25–26, 28–31, 36, 39, 51–52
submission, xv, 25–26, 29–33, 36, 38–39, 42, 73
submission grapplers, 29, 32–33, 39
submissions, 25–26, 29–32, 36, 38
sumai, 4
sumo, xiii, xv, xvii, 1–23, 25–39, 41–43
sumo and MMA fighting stances, 51
sumo diet, 33
sumo elders, 11
sumo fighting stance, 52
sumo ring, 25, 33
sumo wrestler, xiii, xvii, 1, 7, 9–10, 12, 15, 18, 21, 23, 29, 32–33
sumo wrestling, xvii, 1, 7, 12–14, 19, 23, 30, 32–34, 155
sumo's winning moves (kimarite), 1, 4, 10–13, 15, 19, 22–23, 25, 27, 36, 38; in techniques, 43, 53, 60, 68, 73, 82, 90, 106–107, 113, 115, 134, 155
sumostable, 5, 12
superior body contact (controlling the opponent's body), 30–31
supplementary techniques, 43, 53

tachi-ai, 12
tactics, xiii, xv, xvii, 3, 12–14, 17, 23, 33–36, 38–39, 157
takedowns, xv, xvii, 20, 25–27, 29–33, 38–39, 42–44; in techniques, 68, 106, 151, 157
tegumi, 2
teppo, 19
Terao, 18–19, 38
The Gracie Way (Peligro), 38, 156
The Text-Book of Ju-Jutsu as practised in Japan (Uyenishi), 38, 156

thigh-grabbing push down (watashikomi), 104

thigh splits (matawari), 5

three basic fighting styles, 32

throw, 2, 4, 6–7, 10–11, 14, 25, 36, 38; in techniques, 44, 60, 68–76, 78–80, 86, 106–107, 112, 116, 124, 126, 132, 134, 140, 146, 151

throwing techniques (nagete), 68

thrust (tsuki), 10, 14, 16, 19–20, 22, 25, 32, 34, 38; in techniques, 60–62, 64–67, 128

thrust down forward (tsukiotoshi), 128

Tomozuma Stable, 9

traditional belt sumo wrestling

traditional Japanese values, 8

transmission scrolls (texts containing the secrets of the system), 2

triangle choke, 36, 39

triple-attack force out (mitokorozeme), 15; in techniques, 90

tsuppari, 19

Tuli, Teila, 32

twist down (makiotoshi), 10, 35; in techniques, 92, 108, 110, 114, 118, 120, 122, 130

twist-down techniques (hinerite), 106

twisting backward knee trip (kirikaeshi), 86–87

two-handed arm twist down (kainahineri), 110

two-handed head twist down (tokkurinage), 122

Ueshiba, Morihei, 2–3, 155

UFC 1: The Beginning, 32

UFC 129, 36

UFC 157, 36

UFC 84, 36

UFC 98, 36

UFC Hall of Famer, 36

UFC Light Heavyweight title belt

UFC on Fox 4, 36

Ultimate Fighting Championship (UFC), 2, 19, 32, 35–37, 39

unarmed single fight, 26, 30–31

underarm (shitate), 11, 22–23, 27

underarm-forward body drop (tsutaezori), 11

underdog, 1, 37, 39

underdog tactics, 39

underhook, 22–23, 27–29, 36; in techniques, 53, 55–60, 68–69, 74, 82, 86–88, 90, 96, 100–101, 106, 108, 110, 112, 114, 116, 118, 120, 122, 140

underhook technique, 55

under-shoulder swing down (katasukashi), 112

United Kingdom, 34

United States, 34, 155

Uyenishi, Sada Kazu, 38, 156

Wakamatsu Oyakata, sumo coach and elder, 9, 16

waki wo shimeru (to close the armpits), 21

weight divisions, 8–9, 33

Western boxer, 32

Western boxing, 32, 40

Western wrestlers, 33, 39

Western wrestling (folkstyle, freestyle, and Greco-Roman), xvii, 2, 32, 36

Western wrestling's fireman's carry, 2

Wilson, Don, 19

wrestling, xv, xvii, 1–2, 4–5, 7, 11–14, 16–17, 19, 23, 28, 30, 32–34, 36, 38–39, 60, 155

wrestling (folkstyle and Greco-Roman), xv, xvii, 1–2, 4–5, 7, 11–14, 16–17, 19, 23, 28, 30, 32–34, 36, 38–39, 60, 155

wrist grab, 26

yokozuna dohyo-iri (grand champion ring-entering ceremony), 16

About the Author

Andrew Zerling is a black-belt martial artist with over two decades of experience in a variety of styles. His work has appeared in the *Journal of Asian Martial Arts* and *Black Belt Magazine* with Brazilian jiu-jitsu master Renzo Gracie. Andrew's first article with Renzo Gracie, "The Neck: The Grappler's Secret Weapon," was fully featured in the book *The Ultimate Guide to Grappling* published by Black Belt Books. Andrew has also earned a BS in biology from Temple University in Philadelphia and has been a technical writer for the food and drug industry. *Sumo for Mixed Martial Arts: Winning Clinches, Takedowns, and Tactics* is Andrew's first book.

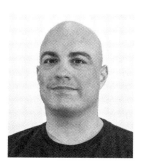

Andrew Zerling resides in Rumson, New Jersey.
www.AndrewZerling.com

BOOKS FROM YMAA

6 HEALING MOVEMENTS
101 REFLECTIONS ON TAI CHI CHUAN
108 INSIGHTS INTO TAI CHI CHUAN
ADVANCING IN TAE KWON DO
ANALYSIS OF SHAOLIN CHIN NA 2ND ED
ANCIENT CHINESE WEAPONS
THE ART AND SCIENCE OF STAFF FIGHTING
ART OF HOJO UNDO
ARTHRITIS RELIEF, 3RD ED.
BACK PAIN RELIEF, 2ND ED.
BAGUAZHANG, 2ND ED.
CARDIO KICKBOXING ELITE
CHIN NA IN GROUND FIGHTING
CHINESE FAST WRESTLING
CHINESE FITNESS
CHINESE TUI NA MASSAGE
CHOJUN
COMPREHENSIVE APPLICATIONS OF SHAOLIN
    CHIN NA
CONFLICT COMMUNICATION
CROCODILE AND THE CRANE: A NOVEL
CUTTING SEASON: A XENON PEARL MARTIAL ARTS THRILLER
DEFENSIVE TACTICS
DESHI: A CONNOR BURKE MARTIAL ARTS THRILLER
DIRTY GROUND
DR. WU'S HEAD MASSAGE
DUKKHA HUNGRY GHOSTS
DUKKHA REVERB
DUKKHA, THE SUFFERING: AN EYE FOR AN EYE
DUKKHA UNLOADED
ENZAN: THE FAR MOUNTAIN, A CONNOR BURKE MARTIAL ARTS
    THRILLER
ESSENCE OF SHAOLIN WHITE CRANE
EXPLORING TAI CHI
FACING VIOLENCE
FIGHT BACK
FIGHT LIKE A PHYSICIST
THE FIGHTER'S BODY
FIGHTER'S FACT BOOK
FIGHTER'S FACT BOOK 2
FIGHTING THE PAIN RESISTANT ATTACKER
FIRST DEFENSE
FORCE DECISIONS: A CITIZENS GUIDE
FOX BORROWS THE TIGER'S AWE
INSIDE TAI CHI
KAGE: THE SHADOW, A CONNOR BURKE MARTIAL ARTS
    THRILLER
KATA AND THE TRANSMISSION OF KNOWLEDGE
KRAV MAGA PROFESSIONAL TACTICS
KRAV MAGA WEAPON DEFENSES
LITTLE BLACK BOOK OF VIOLENCE
LIUHEBAFA FIVE CHARACTER SECRETS
MARTIAL ARTS ATHLETE
MARTIAL ARTS INSTRUCTION
MARTIAL WAY AND ITS VIRTUES
MASK OF THE KING
MEDITATIONS ON VIOLENCE
MERIDIAN QIGONG
MIND/BODY FITNESS
THE MIND INSIDE TAI CHI
THE MIND INSIDE YANG STYLE TAI CHI CHUAN
MUGAI RYU
NATURAL HEALING WITH QIGONG
NORTHERN SHAOLIN SWORD, 2ND ED.
OKINAWA'S COMPLETE KARATE SYSTEM: ISSHIN RYU
POWER BODY

PRINCIPLES OF TRADITIONAL CHINESE MEDICINE
QIGONG FOR HEALTH & MARTIAL ARTS 2ND ED.
QIGONG FOR LIVING
QIGONG FOR TREATING COMMON AILMENTS
QIGONG MASSAGE
QIGONG MEDITATION: EMBRYONIC BREATHING
QIGONG MEDITATION: SMALL CIRCULATION
QIGONG, THE SECRET OF YOUTH: DA MO'S CLASSICS
QUIET TEACHER: A XENON PEARL MARTIAL ARTS THRILLER
RAVEN'S WARRIOR
REDEMPTION
ROOT OF CHINESE QIGONG, 2ND ED.
SCALING FORCE
SENSEI: A CONNOR BURKE MARTIAL ARTS THRILLER
SHIHAN TE: THE BUNKAI OF KATA
SHIN GI TAI: KARATE TRAINING FOR BODY, MIND, AND SPIRIT
SIMPLE CHINESE MEDICINE
SIMPLE QIGONG EXERCISES FOR HEALTH, 3RD ED.
SIMPLIFIED TAI CHI CHUAN, 2ND ED.
SIMPLIFIED TAI CHI FOR BEGINNERS
SOLO TRAINING
SOLO TRAINING 2
SUDDEN DAWN: THE EPIC JOURNEY OF BODHIDHARMA
SUMO FOR MIXED MARTIAL ARTS
SUNRISE TAI CHI
SUNSET TAI CHI
SURVIVING ARMED ASSAULTS
TAE KWON DO: THE KOREAN MARTIAL ART
TAEKWONDO BLACK BELT POOMSAE
TAEKWONDO: A PATH TO EXCELLENCE
TAEKWONDO: ANCIENT WISDOM FOR THE MODERN WARRIOR
TAEKWONDO: DEFENSES AGAINST WEAPONS
TAEKWONDO: SPIRIT AND PRACTICE
TAO OF BIOENERGETICS
TAI CHI BALL QIGONG: FOR HEALTH AND MARTIAL ARTS
TAI CHI BALL WORKOUT FOR BEGINNERS
TAI CHI BOOK
TAI CHI CHIN NA: THE SEIZING ART OF TAI CHI CHUAN, 2ND ED.
TAI CHI CHUAN CLASSICAL YANG STYLE, 2ND ED.
TAI CHI CHUAN MARTIAL APPLICATIONS
TAI CHI CHUAN MARTIAL POWER, 3RD ED.
TAI CHI CONNECTIONS
TAI CHI DYNAMICS
TAI CHI QIGONG, 3RD ED.
TAI CHI SECRETS OF THE ANCIENT MASTERS
TAI CHI SECRETS OF THE WU & LI STYLES
TAI CHI SECRETS OF THE WU STYLE
TAI CHI SECRETS OF THE YANG STYLE
TAI CHI SWORD: CLASSICAL YANG STYLE, 2ND ED.
TAI CHI SWORD FOR BEGINNERS
TAI CHI WALKING
TAIJIQUAN THEORY OF DR. YANG, JWING-MING
TENGU: THE MOUNTAIN GOBLIN, A CONNOR BURKE MARTIAL
    ARTS THRILLER
TIMING IN THE FIGHTING ARTS
TRADITIONAL CHINESE HEALTH SECRETS
TRADITIONAL TAEKWONDO
TRAINING FOR SUDDEN VIOLENCE
WAY OF KATA
WAY OF KENDO AND KENJITSU
WAY OF SANCHIN KATA
WAY TO BLACK BELT
WESTERN HERBS FOR MARTIAL ARTISTS
WILD GOOSE QIGONG
WOMAN'S QIGONG GUIDE
XINGYIQUAN

DVDS FROM YMAA

ADVANCED PRACTICAL CHIN NA IN-DEPTH
ANALYSIS OF SHAOLIN CHIN NA
ATTACK THE ATTACK
BAGUAZHANG: EMEI BAGUAZHANG
CHEN STYLE TAIJIQUAN
CHIN NA IN-DEPTH COURSES 1—4
CHIN NA IN-DEPTH COURSES 5—8
CHIN NA IN-DEPTH COURSES 9—12
FACING VIOLENCE: 7 THINGS A MARTIAL ARTIST MUST KNOW
FIVE ANIMAL SPORTS
JOINT LOCKS
KNIFE DEFENSE: TRADITIONAL TECHNIQUES AGAINST A DAGGER
KUNG FU BODY CONDITIONING 1
KUNG FU BODY CONDITIONING 2
KUNG FU FOR KIDS
KUNG FU FOR TEENS
INFIGHTING
LOGIC OF VIOLENCE
MERIDIAN QIGONG
NEIGONG FOR MARTIAL ARTS
NORTHERN SHAOLIN SWORD : SAN CAI JIAN, KUN WU JIAN, QI MEN JIAN
QIGONG MASSAGE
QIGONG FOR HEALING
QIGONG FOR LONGEVITY
QIGONG FOR WOMEN
SABER FUNDAMENTAL TRAINING
SAI TRAINING AND SEQUENCES
SANCHIN KATA: TRADITIONAL TRAINING FOR KARATE POWER
SHAOLIN KUNG FU FUNDAMENTAL TRAINING: COURSES 1 & 2
SHAOLIN LONG FIST KUNG FU: BASIC SEQUENCES
SHAOLIN LONG FIST KUNG FU: INTERMEDIATE SEQUENCES
SHAOLIN LONG FIST KUNG FU: ADVANCED SEQUENCES 1
SHAOLIN LONG FIST KUNG FU: ADVANCED SEQUENCES 2
SHAOLIN SABER: BASIC SEQUENCES
SHAOLIN STAFF: BASIC SEQUENCES
SHAOLIN WHITE CRANE GONG FU BASIC TRAINING: COURSES 1 & 2
SHAOLIN WHITE CRANE GONG FU BASIC TRAINING: COURSES 3 & 4
SHUAI JIAO: KUNG FU WRESTLING
SIMPLE QIGONG EXERCISES FOR ARTHRITIS RELIEF
SIMPLE QIGONG EXERCISES FOR BACK PAIN RELIEF

SIMPLIFIED TAI CHI CHUAN: 24 & 48 POSTURES
SIMPLIFIED TAI CHI FOR BEGINNERS 48
SUNRISE TAI CHI
SUNSET TAI CHI
SWORD: FUNDAMENTAL TRAINING
TAEKWONDO KORYO POOMSAE
TAI CHI BALL QIGONG: COURSES 1 & 2
TAI CHI BALL QIGONG: COURSES 3 & 4
TAI CHI BALL WORKOUT FOR BEGINNERS
TAI CHI CHUAN CLASSICAL YANG STYLE
TAI CHI CONNECTIONS
TAI CHI ENERGY PATTERNS
TAI CHI FIGHTING SET
TAI CHI FIT FLOW
TAI CHI FIT STRENGTH
TAI CHI FOR WOMEN
TAI CHI PUSHING HANDS: COURSES 1 & 2
TAI CHI PUSHING HANDS: COURSES 3 & 4
TAI CHI SWORD: CLASSICAL YANG STYLE
TAI CHI SWORD FOR BEGINNERS
TAI CHI SYMBOL: YIN YANG STICKING HANDS
TAIJI & SHAOLIN STAFF: FUNDAMENTAL TRAINING
TAIJI CHIN NA IN-DEPTH
TAIJI 37 POSTURES MARTIAL APPLICATIONS
TAIJI SABER CLASSICAL YANG STYLE
TAIJI WRESTLING
TRAINING FOR SUDDEN VIOLENCE
UNDERSTANDING QIGONG 1: WHAT IS QI? • HUMAN QI CIRCULATORY SYSTEM
UNDERSTANDING QIGONG 2: KEY POINTS • QIGONG BREATHING
UNDERSTANDING QIGONG 3: EMBRYONIC BREATHING
UNDERSTANDING QIGONG 4: FOUR SEASONS QIGONG
UNDERSTANDING QIGONG 5: SMALL CIRCULATION
UNDERSTANDING QIGONG 6: MARTIAL QIGONG BREATHING
WHITE CRANE HARD & SOFT QIGONG
WUDANG KUNG FU: FUNDAMENTAL TRAINING
WUDANG SWORD
WUDANG TAIJIQUAN
XINGYIQUAN
YANG TAI CHI FOR BEGINNERS
YMAA 25 YEAR ANNIVERSARY DVD

more products available from . . .
YMAA Publication Center, Inc. 楊氏東方文化出版中心
1-800-669-8892 • info@ymaa.com • www.ymaa.com